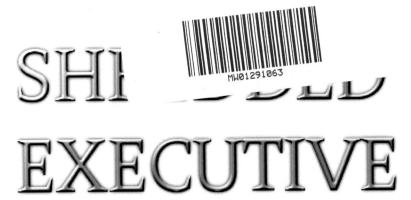

SHREDDED EXECUTIVE

GET SHREDDED, 3 PHASE NUTRITION AND TRAINING PROGRAM AND LIFESTYLE SECRETS FOR THE BUSY PROFESSIONAL

By Daymond Sewall

Daymond Sewall
www.ShreddedExec.com
Laguna Niguel, California

.

Shredded Executive/ Daymond Sewall. —1st ed.
ISBN-10: 1523992700

Contents

Acknowledgments

I don't know where to start because I am truly thankful for every experience, positive or negative, because they have all taught me valuable lessons. I am also truly grateful for all of the people in my life who have helped me, inspired me, educated me, and supported me on my way to a meaningful and impactful life. It would be a book all in itself to thank everyone who has been an integral part of my success in life, but I am going to name the big ones.

My Mom has shaped the man that I am today. Even though I grew up without my father in my life, and was raised by a single mother working multiple jobs, and raising two kids, the one thing that was never in short supply was love. My mom didn't have much to give in material things, money, gifts, but she was always full of love, respect, and guidance. Growing up poor was also what sparked my HUSTLE to become successful in life. Even though I didn't have the father figure to teach me how to be a man, or the guy things, my mom did her best to do so. She instilled in me at a very young age to believe in myself, that I could do anything I wanted, all I had to do was put my mind to it. She also indirectly taught me insane work ethic, by always working 2-3 jobs to make ends meet. So even though as a kid I always felt like I didn't have what I wanted, I never had all the cool things, toys, clothes, or got to do some of the things other kids got to do because we didn't have the money to, I am truly thankful for growing up the way I did because it made me BETTER. Thank you for everything you have done, I truly appreciate it. I love you.

My uncle Jim is like my mothers younger brother, and like my big brother. Because I didn't have a father figure growing up, my uncle Jim was the one who kind of took on the role of teaching me all the guy stuff. Hes the one that bought me my first porn mag, taught me about women, was always there for questions, taught me how to play sports, and he is also the one that introduced me to lifting weights when I was just 8 years old. From that moment on I was hooked! So really you can thank him for this book, because had he not taught me that as a kid, I wouldn't be where I am today. So uncle Jim, I thank you, I know I tell you often, but it is you who has guided me in the direction that I am in now. I truly thank you. I love you bro.

My wife Desiree Sewall, she is one of the most loving, caring people I have ever known. Always has my back, always supports all my crazy dreams, desires, goals, and has put up with my 1000's of hours over years invested in writing this book. When I say crazy dreams, I mean crazy! My work ethic is insanity, and when I am working on achieving a goal I tweak out on it for hours, days, weeks, months, like this book, until it is completed. So thank you for always being so supportive, I am truly grateful for everything that you do for me and the boys. Like I tell you all the time "You are the most loved woman in the world".

To my clients, I truly thank you all. Thank you for being so awesome, so open minded, so fun, and being the faces that have inspired 1,000's around the world. You are part of this process, and how this system, these methods were developed from over a decade of experiences with you. It is the lessons we have learned together that has created this systematic way of getting shredded. So thank you!

"When you want to succeed as bad as you want to breathe, then you will be successful"
-Eric Thomas

Disclaimer

While every effort has been made to ensure the information in this book is correct, you should consult a healthcare professional before undertaking any diet or exercise regime. Aesthetic Lifestyle is not for everyone, and while most of the information in this book is considered to be backed by scientific research and personal experiences, Aesthetic Lifestyles are constantly evolving and over time, some theories may be discredited or improved upon. For this reason, no guarantees can be given in regards to results. No liability is assumed by The Shredded Executive, the person, trademark, or management agency, and all use of this information is the responsibility of the individual.

Introduction

"I'm not going to tell you what you want to hear,
I'm telling you what you NEED to hear."
-Daymond Sewall

Thank you for purchasing *Shredded Executive*. I hope you're ready to get shredded and become more successful! I assure you this book will not be like any book you have ever read, and I am going to talk about things in a way that you've probably never heard before. I might say things that are going to offend you, piss you off, make you question your beliefs, and it's going to change your normal thought patterns. GOOD! Oftentimes, the things you don't want to hear are the things you NEED to hear the most.

I'm not here to blow smoke up your ass and tell you that you're doing everything right and that you're great. I'm not here to be your friend, I created this book to help you live a better, get you shredded, improve your life, and even make you wealthier. I created this book to cut through all the BS misinformation out there and to give you the raw nuts and bolts you need to get SHREDDED. I created this book to help you become a high achiever in all areas of your life! I wrote this book to help you thrive in your life as an entrepreneur, a parent, a spouse, partner, a professional, and as a leader. To make you the BEST version of you aesthetically, and in all areas of your life.

"The worst thing you could be is average."
–Arnold Schwarzenegger

The worst thing in life is being average, living with regret, the "I wish I would have...but..." feeling, and if I can help you get a shredded physique, elevate your confidence, improve your life, improve your relationships, increase your wealth, then I have done my job.

I want to help you elevate your results in the gym and in life. I want you SHREDDED year round. I want you to be turning heads every time you walk into the gym, enter a room, hang out at the pool, or the walk on the beach. I want you feeling proud, confident and accomplished when you look in the mirror. I want your spouse/partner looking at you with those eyes of extreme sexual attraction every time they see you. Yeah, you know those eyes I'm talking about, the ones that say I want to tear your clothes off right now!

But along with the aesthetics I want you to achieve, I want you rich in ALL areas of your life. I love training entrepreneurs, executives, ambitious people, and I have found that it is very, very common for my clients to double, triple, and quadruple their income when they are developing their physique. I have even had clients increase their income over ten-fold!

How is that? Simple, because the person you MUST become to achieve a shredded physique is two times, four times, or even 10 times BETTER than the person you were before. More self-confidence, more self-discipline, and more belief in yourself is developed throughout this process. This transfers to your business, finances, and your relationships.

Your MINDSET is going to improve, the choices you make are going to improve, the actions you take are going to improve, the happiness with YOURSELF is going to improve and the BELIEF in yourself is going to improve. While reading this book you are going to start seeing the world from a completely different lens than you are now. The way you see things, the way you think, the choices you make, are all about to change. You are going to improve vastly from the inside, which is what changes the outside.

"The distance between your dreams and reality is called ACTION."
-Unknown

But here is the catch, YOU MUST TAKE ACTION. Now the fact that you're even reading this book already tells me that you ARE an action taker, but in order for any of these principles, tactics, strategies to work, you have to take action. I mean DAILY, consistent, obsessive, abnormal, action. I call this DTFW a/k/a Do The Fuvking Work! Remember that acronym because you are going to see it consistently throughout this book. It's one of my well known mantras.

It has been said that only 5% of people actually use what they have learned from books, seminars, and conferences. Why is that? Because inspiration is short lived, inspiration will only motivate you so far. We take this up multiple levels higher. In this book, we are focusing on establishing HABITS. Habits are thousands of times stronger than any desire. So when I say DO IT NOW or DTFW, I mean take ACTION NOW, stop reading and DO IT NOW. This book is written step-by-step to program your mind for success, to help you succeed in getting shredded, to help you succeed in improving the quality of your life.

I have read hundreds of books, thousands of scientific articles, on personal development, business, fitness, mindset, nutrition, and I have taken the VERY best, most effective information from these and input them into this book. Over the years, I have realized that there are NO books that offer the kind of mindset, nutrition, and training advice that I give my clients.

The things I teach are YEARS ahead of the average fitness pro, and I am about to change the face of the industry with this book. Because I KNOW that Fit Pros will be purchasing this book and implementing these methods as well, because the proof is in the pudding. My social media following has seen a lot of the insane transformations that my clients have had. The moms with three to five kids, and six-packs. The guys over 50 who are shredded. The incredibly FAST transformations that we have in our gym using these exact strategies. So I KNOW, your trainer, trainers all over the world will also be reading this book to find out my secrets.

I am okay with that, because my intent is to change the WORLD, and the more people I have teaching these methods, using these methods, creates a ripple effect around the world. The ripple effect will create MORE fit, SHREDDED, and RICH men around walking the Earth.

"If you want something you've never had, you've got to do something you've never done." -Thomas Jefferson

I have set out to create a book that just gives the essential tools you need to succeed. But understand, a lot of what you are about to read is probably going to be different than everything you have read or are going to hear elsewhere. That's because a lot of what you are reading, or hearing anywhere else is probably OUTDATED. A lot of the things you will hear are old school methods, methods that have since been debunked, proven ineffective, or just aren't near as effective as what I'm going to teach you in this book. You are going to hear, read, see contradictory info everywhere you look. So ignore EVERYTHING you see that doesn't validate what I'm teaching you. Only listen to one person. You have to stick to the plan for it to be effective.

Also, keep in mind that much of what you read online, via books and articles, is written by bodybuilders/athletes/models that are NOT natural. Meaning they are using steroids, growth hormones, diuretics, and other performance enhancing drugs. I would estimate that 98% or more, of the people you see on social media, magazines, and stages are drug users. Most of the most popular bodybuilders, fitness models, and ripped physiques on social media did NOT attain those physiques naturally.

The methods they teach will NOT be as effective, if even effective at all for you. They didn't earn those physiques through pure nutrition and training; they earned it by taking the drugs. What I am teaching you is to be done DRUG FREE, 100% natural, no hormones, snake oils, potions or cheating. I'm giving you the secrets and success hacks to get you there the fastest route possible, but 100% natural. You are going to develop and EARN your body with the pride and confidence that comes with it.

I want you to forget anything that you have ever heard about nutrition and training, forget anything you have ever read, ever heard, and open your mind. Wipe the slate clean and make it a sponge. ABSORB the information, the strategies, and the methods I'm going to teach you. All of these things you are going to learn are SCIENTIFICALLY PROVEN, EXPERIENCE PROVEN, and WORK EVERY Fuvking time. I GUARANTEE you these methods, systems, strategies will work!

The things I am writing in this book are the exact things I teach my clients on a daily basis that delivers SHREDDED physiques ALL THE TIME. It works! I am the six-pack specialist. I am the Definition Master. Through my years of training clients I have developed a system that ANYONE can implement and they will get ripped. Starting from a beginner level, establishing basic fundamental habits, then progressing as the habits and body progresses. Men, women, young, old, it doesn't matter, the system WORKS!

These results ARE attainable and YES you can achieve this. But you have to be part of the 5% that TAKES ACTION. Like I said earlier, you MUST TAKE ACTION. You MUST DTFW in order for it to work.

So this is enough talk, let's get to work. Get a pen and paper, write the date on the top, and get ready to follow directions. Go, DO IT NOW!

"Do as directed and you are going to LOOK, LIVE, and FEEL better than you have ever expected."
–Daymond Sewall

?

ABOUT THE AUTHOR

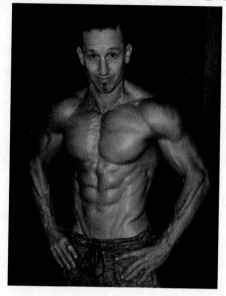

This book is about YOU, YOUR results, YOUR future, YOUR physique, YOUR life, and YOUR income. But I want you to know WHO I am, why I can help you, and how this book came about. So you know why I am writing this, but WHO am I?

My name is Daymond Sewall, I am the owner of three fitness businesses, national level Mens Physique competitor, Winner of a reality TV show, America's Choice Winner of Man of the Year contest, and the father of four boys. I am so serious and obsessed about getting people shredded, I even named my fourth son ABS. Axel Braden Sewall – yep, I sure did. My wife had ABS the entire time she was pregnant.

"The first to help you up are the ones that know how it feels to fall down." –from Action for Happiness

Although I am the six-pack specialist, I have not always been fit. I have been out of shape before, so I know how it feels not to feel comfortable in your own body. I was once out of shape, unhealthy, lethargic, and truly lacking self-confidence. I want you to understand that I KNOW exactly how it feels to be fat, feel fat, to not feel confident shirtless. I know what it feels like to have a gut, muffin top, no abs, no definition and to feel fat. I know exactly what it feels like to feel inferior, insecure and like you're not good enough. I've been there.

When I hit my rock bottom that was the moment in my life where I said, "WTF! Oh, hell no! I refuse to be any less than I know that I am capable." I began to research, change, learn about nutrition, training, started transforming my body, got ripped, and I have NEVER looked back. I became certified as a personal trainer and started teaching others how to do the same. I've been mastering the system of getting ripped and shredded ever since.

The way I felt back then, and the way I feel now being shredded year-round is night and day. This is why I am obsessed about creating SHREDDED physiques for others all around the world. Over the years, I have accumulated numerous personal training certifications (few from NASM, few from NESTA, few others). I have about 13 years of experience in this industry, train physique competitors, am a competitor myself, and I personally live SHREDDED year round. I LIVE by example. I lead from the front. Everything I am going to teach you, I DO myself. The training methods, and nutritional strategies, you are going to learn in this book I do myself, as well as teach all of my clients the same tactics. I am always leading by example.

"A smart man learns from his mistakes. A wise man learns from the mistakes of others." –Otto von Bismarck

I have already made all of the mistakes, I have tried all the different types of training, diets strategies, I have failed, I have made bad choices, I have utilized the methods that were once taught that are now outdated. But through this process, through these failures, through these mistakes, I have found what works. I have discovered what is the easiest, fastest route, the most effective strategies, and developed a systematic way of implementing it. This book is what I feel is the BEST of the BEST. Utilizing these strategies, I have succeeded, and I have helped countless others do the same. This system I developed works EVERY SINGLE TIME. For every single person who follows the plan.

The things I am teaching you are from years and years in the trenches, years and years of trial and error, years and years of researching, learning, reading, and implementing. Everything I am going to teach you are truly success hacks! If you're in business, I KNOW you appreciate hacks. I know you appreciate just getting straight to the point to produce the results. That's what this book is all about creating the shortest possible route from where you are, to where you want to be, and then how to KEEP it and still live and enjoy your life.

I live and breathe this lifestyle. The reason I am writing this book is because I truly want to help YOU finally and permanently get the physique you deserve. The fact that you purchased this book is proof enough that you are ready to take action to get SHREDDED. I commend you for taking the first step. Thank you for your purchase.

I will be covering the most crucial elements you need to succeed, many of which are valuable elements that seem to be missing from most fitness books. Elements like training your mindset, goal setting, nutrition, training, and even throw in some lifestyle hacks throughout.

Unlike most magazines and articles, this is NOT going to be some kind of gimmicky marketing ploy to get you to buy supplements or other products. This is not going to be some complex literature on science that is over your head. It is designed to develop your mind and your body step-by-step to success: getting shredded, simplified.

This book is going to cut through the confusion and misinformation that is taught today. My intent is to teach you step by step how to get a SHREDDED physique and KEEP it. EVERYTHING you need to know about getting SHREDDED and staying SHREDDED is included in this book. EVERYTHING.

Some of the things you're going to hear over and over throughout the book as the pieces start coming together. This is intentional, this is to educate you, inform you, remind you, so you RETAIN the information. The more you see it, the more you read it, the more you REMEMBER it.

If you are more experienced and have been training and dieting, this guide will show you how to do it right, and do it better. You are going to be walking around shredded all year! This book is setup step-by-step, so please do NOT skip around. Go through each chapter, follow the directions, and DTFW (Do the fuvking work.)

There is a reason WHY we do what we do. Everything in this program is designed in order to make you a success. If at any time you feel lost, confused or don't understand something, REREAD the previous paragraph or chapter. This book is written as SIMPLE as possible for easy comprehension, but if you are new to this lifestyle you may need to reread some portions. As soon as you get done reading the entire book, read it again three to five more times.

Why? Because each time that you read it you're going to learn something new. You're going to pick up something you may have forgotten already, or learn something you may have just missed the first time. Things will start to make more sense. You will be in a better place each time, so what you absorb will build upon the last. The more you read it, the more you learn, the more you retain, the more confident you feel with your actions. So read it over, and over, and over. I recommend one chapter per day, either first thing in the morning or right before bed. Deal or deal? Good!

Get a pen and keep index cards or paper handy, and TAKE notes. One of the BEST ways to learn, is to learn with the INTENT to be able to TEACH someone else. If you don't understand it enough to teach another, you don't understand it well enough. So READ with the intent to TEACH and you will grasp all of the information I am about to teach you. The results are worth the EFFORT.

"The difference between dreamers and achievers is called ACTION."
-James Arthur Ray

You are going to have to DO something with this program to make it work for you. You must ACTUALLY do what I tell you to do. DTFW and take the actions and it WILL happen. The results are going to be phenomenal. The person you become is going to be life changing. But this takes ACTION, so DTFW. (Do the fuvking work!)

I have helped countless people around the world get SHREDED and in that process made them more wealthy. The discipline, self-confidence, and belief in yourself you are going to acquire from getting SHREDDED, is going to elevate your success in business and increase your income. I want you to become another one of my success stories: shredded and successful.

Let's start by picking a date 90 days from now, mark it on your calendar, then six months from now, mark it on your calendar. Use either your phone, planner, or calendar on your desk or wall. By the 90-day mark you are either going to be SHREDDED already or getting close to it. Six months from now, you should be LIVING the lifestyle, living SHREDDED and you should notice your income, relationships, and life drastically improved.

Today, I want you to write down a few things so we have a record of your starting point. On your index cards, or notepad answer these questions:

1. How you feel about your body today? How is it rated on a scale of 1-10?
2. What does your current physique hold you back from?
3. How is your energy throughout the day? How is it on a scale 1-10?
4. How are your finances? 1-10?
5. How is your relationship? 1-10?
6. How is your income? 1-10? How much are you making?
7. How is your overall happiness in life? 1-10?
8. How much do you weigh?
9. What is your waist size (around the belly button)?

10. What do you feel you look like today? (fat, gross)

Date this card and keep it because in the future I want you to look back on these and ask yourself the same questions.

Now go take your shirt off and go take a selfie on your phone and email it to yourself, save it on computer. You will WANT to see the progress weekly and have a record of where you started from. Your transformation is going to be incredible and the only way you'll see the magnitude of how great it is if you have a starting point. So GO take the picture, now! DTFW!

So by now what should you have done? I'm testing you to see if you are an action taker. You should have a before pic and you should have written the answers to these questions down. We need a record of your starting point. The reason I am asking you this and having you write this down is so (1) you create awareness of what needs work and improvement, (2) so you have a record of how you are TODAY. In 90 days, I want you to reassess where you are, then again in six months I want you to reassess.

"All winners are trackers." –Darren Hardy

Winners track everything. So track where you start, create awareness on areas you need to improve, track to assess and improve. Remember that quote above, because you are going to see examples of this throughout the book. I have helped many people get SHREDDED physiques, and through that process have helped many people increase their wealth, and create extraordinarily successful lives. There is only ONE real success, and that is to be able to live your life on YOUR terms, how you want, looking the way you want, feeling the way you want, and with the lifestyle you want.

This process is NOT going to be easy, as matter of fact, its sometimes going to really suck. But I assure you every drop of sweat, every uncomfortable moment, every grunting rep, every invested minute, every ounce of effort you put in WILL pay off, it WILL be worth it. It's the pain from the effort, discipline, and sacrifice, that makes the success so much more glorious. So expect to be constantly uncomfortable, it's through our toughest times, the our true success is developed.

As an entrepreneur myself, I know that TIME is our most valuable commodity. I also know that the majority of high-achieving successful entrepreneurs prioritize their health and themselves because they know it will increase their wealth. From having the energy to hustle and focus consistently, stress relief, endorphin high to process thoughts more clearly, to improving their aesthetics so they feel better about themselves.

Most highly successful entrepreneurs KNOW that their bodies and their HEALTH is the key to their productivity, energy, success, longevity, and wealth. This is why most of these people live very active lifestyles. This book is for those that want to be high achieving executives/entrepreneurs that also want to look incredible.

Get a pen and paper so you can complete the next few steps and take notes. Taking notes helps your brain retain the information. Retention of this knowledge is key. Go DO IT NOW. Pen, paper! Remember, for this to work you must take ACTION. You must DTFW!

Let's do this!!!

[2]

Know Your Why

"He who has a WHY can endure any how."
–Friedrich Nietzsche

Want to know one of the main reasons why you lose your motivation? Because you have never invested the time and effort into your MENTAL game. This journey of getting shredded abs is a MENTAL game. What did I just say? This journey of getting ripped is a MENTAL game.

It's more mental than physical. Learn to control your thoughts, and you control your choice, decisions, actions, and behaviors. This ultimately leads to control over your results.

One of the biggest reasons why you have lost steam, lost motivation in the past, and haven't created the body you want is because you haven't been clear on your WHY. The only way you are going to be able to stick to the program, stay committed, stay dedicated to this process is if you know your "WHY." The "Why" is the REAL reason, the driving force behind your desire to change, get shredded, reveal your six-pack. You can ONLY change if your WHY is so important, so powerful, so clear in your mind, that NOTHING will stop you from achieving it.

Your WHY is what is going to make you get in the gym when you are tired. It's going to make you wake up at 4:00 a.m. to go train before starting your day. It's going to make you be disciplined with your nutrition. It's going to make you do the work that is required to achieve the body that you want. So take some time and figure out your true WHY.

What do you want to achieve? Why?

Why do you want abs?

Why do you want to be SHREDDED?

Why is being shredded so important to you?

What is being shredded going to do for you?

Why is it important for you to be able to do this?

How is your life going to change from achieving a shredded physique?

What do you want to be experiencing that you're not now?

There isn't a wrong answer, it just needs to have meaning and a purpose to YOU. It doesn't matter what other people think, it doesn't matter how shallow it is, it doesn't matter how vain it is, the only thing that matters is that it's IMPORTANT to you and fuels your motivation. This is what will drive you, this is what is going to CHANGE YOU.

We are emotional animals and focusing on the emotional reasons why you want to achieve your goal will propel you forward. Once you get clear on your WHY you will find solutions to your challenges, you will start doing the work, you will do MORE than you ever have, you will start prioritizing the things that matter that will deliver RESULTS.

Do you want to look ripped on vacation? Why?
Do you want to compete in a physique contest? Why?
Do you want to post your pics on social media? Why?
Are you getting ready for a photoshoot? Why?
Do you want to feel good about your body and increase your confidence?
Do you want to be and feel more sexually attractive?
Do you want to lead by example for your kids? Why?
Do you want to prove that you can do it? Why?
Do you want to be able to feel confident at the beach?

Whatever your reason, this is going to be the driving force behind your actions.

So take some time, figure it out, put it in writing! Your why creates motion, which will put you *into* motion. Think about the real reason WHY you want this, and put it down on paper, there is a magic that happens when you put something that's in your mind down in writing.

What is your WHY?

Just like the German philosopher Frederick Nietzsche once said, "He who has a WHY can endure any how." Knowing your why is an important first step in figuring out HOW to achieve the goals you are striving to achieve. When you know your why, you will find the courage, motivation, put in the work needed to get ahead.

What is it deep down inside that motivates you to take action to get this shredded physique? What is the driving force behind this desire? Write it down and keep it on your mind at all times. It could be more confidence, vacation, leading by example for kids, to feel better, etc. Your why is YOUR why. What moves you is the only thing that matters. Knowing your why is an important first step into figuring out HOW to achieve your goals. Only when you know WHY will you find the courage, motivation, to do the work needed to accomplish your goal. Only when you know WHY will you stay motivated when the times get tough and the challenges are rough.

Take some time and write down 10-20 reasons WHY you want to be shredded, WHY it's important to you. Why do you want to get shredded? Why is it important? Write it down, because it's important that you know the DEEP rooted reasons WHY you want the body you want.

1._____
2._____
3._____
4._____
5._____
6._____
7._____
8._____
9._____
10._____

Now that you have down your WHY, let's move to the next step. But first, let's review:

1. This journey of getting shredded is a _____ game?
2. What is one of the main reasons you have lost motivation in the past?
3. What does knowing your why do?
4. What does the famous quote by Frederick Nietzsche once "He who has a WHY can endure any how" mean to you?

5. What do you think is YOUR most powerful WHY? Which one motivates you or moves you the most?

6. Why is it important that we identify and establish your why?

[3]

Developing a Shredded Executive Mindset

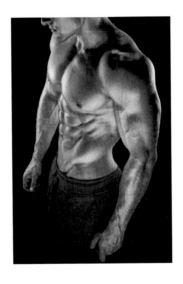

In this chapter, we are going to talk about the mindset you need to have to succeed in this journey. We are going to discuss goal setting, the power of the mind, and some of the actions steps needed to achieve the shredded physique you have always wanted.

"Setting goals is the first step in turning the invisible into the visible."
- Tony Robbins

Goal setting by definition is a powerful process for thinking about your ideal future, and for motivating yourself to turn this vision of this future into reality. We all know setting goals are very important, but what do you think is one of the most overlooked things when it comes to you achieving your goal of getting shredded? One of the most overlooked, underestimated tricks to achieving any goal, is putting it in writing.

"Writing down your goals, specifically, increases your chances of achieving them by 1,000%." – Brian Tracy

This always amazes me, the fact that we all know intuitively that those why write down their goals accomplish SIGNIFICANTLY more than those who do not, yet most people do not do this. Like Brian Tracy says, writing down your goals increases your chances of achieving them by 1,000! This is something that I have found most execs do for business, finances, sales, appointments, closes, but when it comes to their physique its almost unheard of. You achieve your business goals by setting goals, tracking numbers, using deadlines, but aren't doing it for your body? Really?

The human mind is the human mind, and it is a goal-seeking organism. Give it targets, and it will work its ass off to achieve it. Whether that is in business, finances, relationships, or getting shredded. Most people think that just having it in the mind is good enough, but as you know in business you need to have your goals in writing, everything tracked, accounted for, visible and always focused on reaching your daily, weekly, monthly targets. Achieving success with your physique is exactly the same.

If you are one of these people that think "I know what I want, I don't need to write it down". Really? How has that been working for you? Are you shredded yet? Got the perfect body yet? If you're reading this, then probably not, and part of the reason is because you haven't created a CLEAR goal with CLEAR daily action steps to achieve it.

So are you tired of just "knowing" and ready to finally succeed? Then it's time to step your game up and DTFW(Do the fuvking work).

Your current goal hasn't been specific enough, hasn't been clear enough, hasn't had any urgency, which is why you haven't achieved it. You set financial goals for business don't you? Yes. If you have a goal to achieve $1 Million or even $100 Million, you have that goal set right? Yes. You probably even have a date or timeline for exactly WHEN you want to achieve it, right? Yes. You probably know exactly what you need to do each day, each week, each month in business to hit these goals, right? Yes or yes?

Well guess what? When it comes to having a million-dollar body, it works the same way. When you write something down, you are stating your INTENTION and setting things in motion. When you put pen to paper, it goes from just an idea, a wish, a thought, to A COMMITMENT.

The practice of goal setting not only accelerates your success, it is also a prerequisite for happiness. You are here because you want to get shredded, you want to look awesome and feel awesome, you want to have incredible confidence and feel sexually attractive right? Of course.

What do these things do for you? They increase HAPPINESS in your life, right? Psychologists tell us that people who make consistent progress towards meaningful goals live happier more satisfied lives than those who don't. So what does that tell you? If you want to live a happier, more satisfied, confident life, then you need to do what? Make progress towards meaningful goals! Make progress on getting shredded!

Are you sold on why this is so important? Awesome! Now get your pen and paper and lets do this! I'm going to cut through and get straight to the point, entire books have been written on this topic, although this is a vital key to your success I want to get you moving forward ASAP. I'm just going to give you the hacks.

Setting Powerful Goals in 3 Easy Steps

Step #1: Be Specific

You have to have a clear, specific TARGET, with daily processes and a deadline to achieve it by. Laser guided coordinates for your missile to hit its target.

- -How many pounds do you want to lose?
- -What do you want your waist size to be?
- -What does your ideal physique look like?
- -When you think about the perfect version of you, what do you look like?
- -What size are your arms, chest, calves, etc.?
- -Who do you want to look like?
- -What is your ideal weight and body fat %?
- -What will it feel like to walk around with that physique?

- -What will you feel like in this new body?

The human mind is a goal-seeking organism, give it a target, that is clear, concise and has a deadline to achieve it by and it will work its ass off to achieve it. But that's ONLY if the coordinates are clear and concise.

Your current goal of "I want to get abs" (weak, boring and not motivating) becomes, "I am shredded, 175 lb., 5% body fat, with a six-pack and a 28-inch waist by December 31, 2016." See the difference?

If two execs had goals, Exec #1, that just had the thought, "I want to get abs?" and Exec #2, had a written goal of, "I am ripped, 175 lb., 5% body fat, with a six-pack and a 28-inch waist by December 31, 2016," who do you think is going to achieve their goal the quickest?

Exec #2 Right? Sounds obvious, yet most people don't do this, which is why most people don't have abs and live in the body they want. It sounds obvious that if this is your goal, that's what you should be doing, right?

Then why haven't you?

The goal that is specific, that is detailed, that creates an image in your mind that creates urgency, and is the goal that is MOTIVATING. That is how you set physique goals. You set your physique goals very much like you set your business domination goals.

Step #2: Be Committed

Have you set goals in the past yet continue failing reaching them? Have you tried affirmations and but still not getting the results you want? Want to know why?

Well, there are probably many reasons why, from lack of clarity, lack of urgency, lack of specificity, but there is one main thing that I want to discuss here that is probably the real reason why you aren't where you want to be. That one thing is COMMITMENT.

Writing down a goal is great but it's not enough. So just saying, "I am shredded, 175 lb., 5% body fat, with a six-pack and a 28 inch waist by December 31st 2016" is great, it's the first step, but it can be made even BETTER! Your goal and focus can be dialed-in and made MORE laser focused if you do one thing. Want to know what that is?

That one thing is making COMMITMENTS! Your goal should be rephrased and begin with the words "I am 'committed' to...."

> **"I AM are two of the most powerful words, for**
> **you put after them shapes your reality."**
> **–Anonymous quote**

The words "I am" are powerful, whatever follows these words starts the creation of it.

Why? Because the words "I am" precede the subconscious beliefs that you program yourself with. "I am" is often followed by a belief, that belief creates actions, decisions, behaviors and ultimately what you achieve. Think of these two words as a COMMAND.

> **"I am the greatest!" –Muhammad Ali**

Then follow your "I am" with the words "committed to..." to make your goal a command that you are DEDICATED to. So "I am shredded, 175 lb., 5% body fat, with a six-pack and a 28-inch waist by December 31st 2016," gets one little tweak:

"I am COMMITTED to being shredded, 175 lb., 5% body fat, with a six-pack and a 28-inch waist by December 31st 2016."

Now doesn't that sound and feel so much more powerful? You may even feel a little anxiety just reading and writing this, GOOD! That uncomfortable feeling is your sign you are stepping outside your comfort zone and growing.

Step #3: Be Committed To Actions!

Now the next part of achieving your goals requires your COMMITMENT to taking the daily actions to achieve them. Once you create a goal that is specific, a goal that is a commitment, then you break it down into ACTIONS. Your commitment to your goal is reinforced by making the small daily commitments, actions, or habit that is required for your goal to become your REAL outcome.

Simply put, make a commanded commitment (big goal), then follow it by the action steps (small goals) that you need to achieve it.

"Focus on the process and the results will come." - Unknown

The process of you getting shredded comes from the daily actions, daily goals, daily activities, and daily habits that are required for you to achieve the shredded physique you seek. These daily actions are what will deliver your results by the date you set. So, what do you need to do each day to achieve your goal by that date? What things must you do DAILY that are going to make the biggest impact, that will make you progress day after day? What do you need to do on a daily basis to shredded day after day?

We need to create a few daily actions (processes) that if done daily, will take you exactly where you want to be.

You need about three to five (or more) things that you are going to need to do DAILY in order to achieve this. I'm going to get this ball rolling for you and just tell you the basic fundamentals you'll need to succeed. You will need to specify, personalize and improve these later, but for now, put down these 5 things you MUST do to achieve this goal. If you're like the normal person you're going to need these basics, but feel free to update, add more, or put it in your own words. I'm just giving you the hacks. ;)

Write these five things down. I want to plant the seed in your mind what it's going to take to succeed getting shredded. So DTFW put pen to paper now.

"We are what we repeatedly do. Excellence then, is not an act, but a habit."
-Aristotle

Get Shredded Hack List:

1. I am committed to training in the gym seven days a week. (Yes, seven days. I will explain below.)
2. I am committed to eating healthy, hitting my calories and macros (pro, carbs, fats) and staying on point seven days a week.(recommendations coming later)
3. I am committed to drinking 1.5 to over 2 gallons of water per day. (Vital to your success)
4. I am committed to tracking my workouts and my calorie burn goal daily. (you will learn both later)

5. I am committed to being disciplined in social situations, living the fitness lifestyle, staying dedicated and consistent.

Do you see what I did there? We created your goal, then we created five mini-action goals. But did you see what we did with all of them? We made them affirmative COMMITMENTS. We made them subconscious commands. All they need are the specific target numbers to make them more effective. You will get your goal calories, macros, calorie burn goals, and learn how to track workouts later on in this book.

By doing those five things daily, you are GUARANTEED to succeed. So write those and your big goal down daily. Yes, that's a total of six sentences at the minimum. Connect your brain, your hand, to your goal and those five action items. As you read more in this book, you will be able to refine and specify in MORE detail these five things.

Pay attention because as the book progresses, you're going to know exactly what your macros are, and how many calories to eat so you can fill in commitment #2 with the specific numbers to improve the programming and command of the action. You will also learn how to track your workouts, how to find out how many calories you burn during your workouts, and how many calories YOU should burn every workout for commitment #4. You will also learn the tricks on how to socialize the smart way so you stay on track year round. So as this book progresses, so should your commitments that you write daily.

I want you to WRITE those six things (your goal and the five actions) down two times a day at the MINIMUM. Starting NOW, just like how they are, then as you learn more you can specify your target numbers and fine tune these.

Get a notebook and each morning when you wake, get up, write down those six things, your goal and your actions steps. This will program your subconscious mind from the START of the day and keep you focused all day. Then right before bed, write down all six again. While you are sleeping, your mind is processing this information, programming your subconscious mind, and when you wake up you are going to be more focused. You can absolutely do this more than two times per day, but first thing in the morning and before bed are the mandatories.

You can also do this for ALL of your goals, for specific body parts, or other physical, performance goals. For example, let's say you want to deadlift 500 pounds in 12 months, it would look something like this:

"I am committed to being a 500 lb. Deadlifter by Dec 31st 2016. I am committed to deadlifting, three times per week, every week. I am committed to rolling out my muscles, stretching, for 60 minutes daily to keep my body on point. I am committed to training with my powerlifting team each training day, every week. I am committed to eating nutritious foods and supplementing adequately daily to provide the nutrients my body needs to recover from each session."

It works for all goals. Just find out specifically WHAT you want, pick a reasonable deadline that creates urgency, make it a commitment, then figure out what daily actions you need to commit to achieve it. Like I said, I'm just giving you the basic fundamentals. Just remember make them a command, "I AM Committed to...," add deadlines for goals, then frequency for the actions. Simple, huh? You can apply that to business too. You're welcome. Success requires action, so DTFW and program your mind.

Review:

1. Why do most people fail at achieving their goal?
2. What is the first step to setting goals?
3. What is the second step?
4. What is the third step?
5. How many times per day do you need to write them down?

[4]

See Yourself as a Success

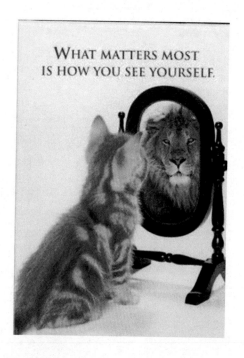

Self-image

We have discussed setting goals and how to make them more effective. Have you noticed we focus a lot on the mentality of getting shredded? Want to know why? This journey of getting shredded is primarily MENTAL. You've got to get shredded in your MIND before you will ever get shredded in life. One of the processes to getting it in your mind is by creating your IDEAL self-image.

Your self-image is simply HOW you see yourself. The image you have of yourself in your mind is ultimately the image you CREATE in your life. Want to know why you self-sabotage? Want to know what why you lose focus and fall off the wagon? Besides not having a clear, specific goal with commitments, one of the main reasons why you have fallen off the wagon and self-sabotaged is because of your self-image.

Your self-image is of the fatter, weaker, softer, undisciplined one. You see yourself as you ARE, or as you recently were. If you are at 200 pounds, working on getting to a shredded 175 pounds, but still have the self-image of you being at 200 pounds, you will soon self-sabotage to go back to 200 pounds.

How you picture yourself is like a target you set for your mind to aim at. How you see yourself is the image that your subconscious will work to create. Did you know that your subconscious is what controls 95-98% of the actions you take daily? It's not only responsible for your breathing, heart rate, emotions and bodily functions, it is also the primary driver of your daily behaviors, daily actions, and your decisions in life, business, relationships, and with your physique. So if you have an image of yourself failing, being fat, being 200 pounds, being soft, being overweight, being undisciplined, being weak, being inconsistent, falling off track, that's EXACTLY the results it will deliver.

According to bestselling author and brain researcher, John Assaraf, your mind is like your home air conditioning unit. Your self-image is like the thermostat in your home set at 70 degrees. Now the way that the control center (the brain) of your thermostat works is it will always work to keep the temperature at 70 degrees. If the temperature rises to 71 or more, the AC kicks on and brings it back down to 70, then it shuts off. If the temperature drops to 69 or below, the heater will kick on and bring it back up to 70 degrees.

Sounds pretty simple, right?

Throughout our childhood, we are programmed and conditioned to believe certain things. All of our beliefs about our true potential in every area of our lives was instilled in us by our parents, teachers, peers, caregivers, books, and experiences we have had. All of these programs are kept in our subconscious mind and operate just like the set temperature of our homes. The image you hold in your mind, the beliefs you keep, is your SET temperature.

This is why every time you have set out to get the body, lose weight, get shredded, you stop, you cheat on your diet, you fall off the wagon, you binge, you miss workouts, you procrastinate, and you make poor choices. The moment you started to deviate from your self-image by losing weight, working out, changing your body, your subconscious kicked in and started to self-sabotage you to deliver the REAL self-image you are keeping in your mind.

It often masks itself by the "I'm too busy" excuse for most execs and people. When your thermostat kicks in your subconscious will make you procrastinate tasks to slow down your productivity, which will make you run out of time to train, validating the "I'm too busy" to train excuse. It will make you miss training sessions. It will do the same when it comes to cooking, preparing meals, so you can justify eating out and making poor choices. These are just two examples of how it kicks in to sabotage you, and bring you back to your personal 70-degree setting.

Make sense? So how do we overcome this?

"What you see is what you create." -Unknown

One of the biggest most important elements to you getting shredded is CREATING a shredded self-image. Creating the image in your mind of the IDEAL body you want, the way you want to feel, and life you want to live. You have to SEE yourself ALREADY having it, you have to visualize it, feel it, affirm it, and imprint this Shredded image in your mind.

This is also WHY I want you writing down your goals two times a day and this is WHY I want you showing up to the gym seven days a week. This is all to create the IMAGE in your mind, and TRAIN your subconscious for success. This is to hack your subconscious mind to develop the shredded self-image so you can become success story.

Do you see how these pieces are starting to fit together now? This book is very strategic; there is a reason why we do everything we do.

If you're like most people, you may have a hard time trying to picture this, especially if you've never had a shredded body. That's okay. There is a hack for this is too, just google an image someone who inspires you, someone that you'd like to look like. Then print out those pictures and place EVERYWHERE. Save one to the desktop of your computer, your phone, place pics on your bathroom mirror, on your fridge, keep one right here on your notebook that you write your goals in. Even on the dashboard of your car.

All throughout the day when you see this image, visualize looking down and seeing those abs on YOUR body. See yourself walking into the gym with a shredded physique turning heads. See yourself developing that body. See yourself training hard, sweating, grunting, burning insane amounts of calories. See yourself standing on the scale at your ideal weight. See yourself eating flawlessly, weighing, tracking your food so you can develop the body you want.

Just like how you picture yourself making $100,000 to $100,000,000 a year, to achieve your business or financial goals, you have to picture yourself living with a million-dollar BODY.

So what does your million-dollar body look like?
What does it feel like to walk around with a body like that?
How is your life going to be different?
How are people going to treat you?
What does a guy who is shredded train like?
What does he eat like?
What does he act like?
How does he behave in social situations?

Think like a shredded guy would think.
Live like a shredded guy lives.
Act like a shredded guy acts.
Train like a shredded guy trains.
Make daily choices like you are ALREADY there.
See yourself as a success! Think like a success! Act like a Success!
Then DTFW and CREATE it.

Review:

1. Why do people self-sabotage?

2. What example did I use to explain how the brain works?
3. What happens if your self-image is of an unfit version?
4. What do you need to do two times a day, to help program and imprint the right self-image?
5. Where are you going to put images of your ideal physique?
6. What do you need to see yourself as?

[5]

How to Become a Morning Person

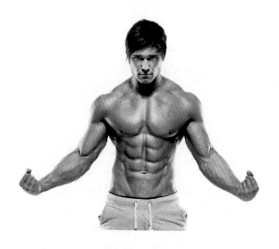

In this chapter, we are going to talk about how to become a morning person. Yes, it's possible, there are tricks to this as well. So pay attention, because this one thing can completely transform your life and give you more time to spend with your family.

What is the number #1 excuse most people give as to why they don't work out? Time. Too busy. Etc. Yes or yes?

We discussed one of the reasons this happens in the last chapter, so let's assume you have that on point now and your self-image is good. If there is truly a time issue there is another way to CREATING more time. There is one thing you could do to eliminate a time issue. This one thing could also help you establish the habit of consistently training daily. This one thing could also accelerate your productivity throughout the day.

What is this one thing?

GTFU earlier! Yes, Get The Fuvk Up Earlier and CREATE more time in your day. If you have a TIME issue, meaning you tend to work late, get stuck on projects, miss training, then you NEED to become a morning person. You need to go get it in BEFORE you start your day. I'm not talking about with your blow up doll, I mean in the gym.

I do a lot of personal development, I study the greats, and with that, I have found that one of the common traits among the MAJORITY of the really high achievers is that they have made a habit of waking up extra early. Not only do they wake up early, one of the first things they do in those early morning is TRAIN.

So if TIME is an issue, but your goal is to be shredded and super successful, then this is something that you are going to have to do. One of the keys to becoming successful in any area of your life is by investing your time wisely. Time is $. Time is opportunity. To develop an incredible physique is going to require discipline, dedication, and consistency. If time is your challenge, early mornings are your solution. Studies prove that those who rise early are more productive and earn more money.

But it's not only about just waking up early, it's HOW you invest their time and WHAT you do in those early morning hours that determines level of your success. If you wake up at

4am and sit on your ass, procrastinate, do nothing productive, obviously you're going to continue to be in the same boat you are currently on in life. But if you get up, train your ass off, start working before the world wakes, you will have exponential results.

The majority of top earning CEO's in the world make a habit of getting up early. Disney CEO Bob Iger wakes up at 4:30 a.m. every morning. Apple CEO Tim Cook wakes up at 4:30 a.m. every morning. Starbucks CEO Howard Schultz wakes up at 4:30 a.m. NBA Brooklyn Nets CEO Brett Yormark gets up at 3:30 a.m. to be at the office by 4:30 a.m. Virgin America CEO David Cush wakes up at 4:15 a.m. Sir Richard Branson wakes up at 5:45 a.m. and trains daily, too.

Some of the most notable actors and athletes also have early rising habits. Kobe Bryant has been known to be IN the gym ALREADY training at 4:00 a.m. Dwayne "The Rock" Johnson gets up at 4:00 a.m. daily to train and is known to get up even earlier to get his training done before shooting for 12 to over 15 hours a day on movies sets.

I cannot think of a single great person in the course of history who did not wake up early to work on their craft. Benjamin Franklin, Winston Churchill, the Dalai Lama, Gandhi, Aristotle, and Buddha all did this, just to name a few more.

Waking up early is one of the hardest habits you will ever develop but becoming successful at it will cause TREMENDOUS benefits. This is one habit that directly impacts the quality of your life and how much you are able to achieve. If being shredded and successful is your goal, then rising early should become your new secret weapon.

"The earlier you wake up, the more you can do when the sun is up."
-Unknown

This habit enables you to do more things during the most productive hours of the day. Why is waking up early so beneficial?

Simply put, the battle of your mind, self-discipline, self-control and self-esteem is won by beating that inner voice that says to stay in bed. When you are in charge of your inner voice, this instills discipline and sends a message to your subconscious that you DO what you intend to do. Winning!

It also creates MORE time, more time to train, more time to plan, and more time to tackle those tough tasks. It's also quiet. Most of us have kids, a box full of emails that can consume an entire day to answer, interruptions from employees, or fires to put out at the office during the day.

So when is the best time to do those important tasks? You guessed it, first thing in the morning. By making this one thing a habit, you get one step ahead of everyone else. Now you see just a few reasons why the super successful are super successful.

How early should you get up? That depends on how much time you want and need. I recommend two to three hours before you are supposed to start your day. Do you want to know how much more time just getting up two hours earlier creates? Two hours earlier daily equates to 730 hours EXTRA per year. This equates to 30 FULL 24-hour days EXTRA. That's 13 FULL months instead of 12 per year!

What could you do with your body if you had an extra two hours a day? What could you do with an extra two hours a day with your business or family? That's two more hours to invest in yourself. Two more hours that give you a jump on your day. Two more hours of uninterrupted time to tackle those important tasks before the rest of the world wakes.

The difference between someone getting up at say 5:00 a.m. and 7:00 a.m. for 40 years, if they go to bed at the same time, is equivalent to an additional 10 years to a man's life. TEN YEARS! How much could you accomplish with 10 extra years?

> *"If you do the work, you get rewarded. There are no shortcuts in life"*
> *– Michael Jordan*

The majority of my most ripped, successful clients are the ones who are early risers. So if you want more shreds and more success, what do you think you need to do? GTFU EARLY! I know what you're thinking: "Holy crap! I'm not a morning person and that's INSANELY early." The majority of the people who say "I'm not a morning person" are also the same majority that are low achievers, broke and out of shape.

The person who says "I'm not a morning person" rarely achieves a shredded physique, or the high levels of success they want to have. "I'm not a morning person" rarely drives a Lamborghini, rarely lives in a mansion, rarely gets to travel the world, and lives a lavish lifestyle.

If success is what you seek, physically, financially, aesthetically, in your relationships and long working hours are truly your issue, then you're going to have to wake up early. You're going to have to do a lot of things that make you uncomfortable, this is just part of success.

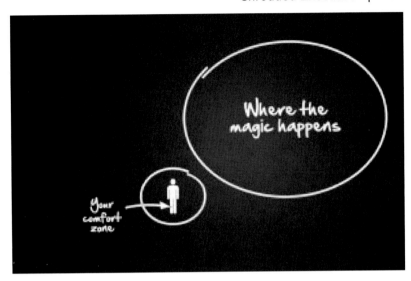

What time do you need to wake up? That really depends on you, how successful you want to be and how much time you need. But I recommend between 4:00 a.m. and 5:30 a.m., seven days a week. I personally wake up at 4:00 a.m. every day. My intent is to be ridiculously successful in the fitness industry and I will do whatever it takes for however long it takes to achieve my goals. World Domination! (Hint, this is the type of mindset you have to have to succeed in getting shredded and become a morning person.)

Now let's get to the tips on how to become a morning person. When does your preparation for waking up early begin? The night before – hell, even days before. It also begins with changing your beliefs, because your beliefs become your experiences.

Believing "I'm not a morning person" is why you're not a morning person. So start instilling the belief of "I love waking up early. I am a morning person. I am COMMITTED to being a morning person." (You may need to add that to your daily commitment list.) Program THIS into your mind and you will start to experience these beliefs.

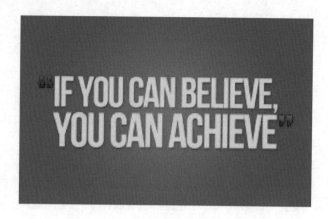

It begins in the mind. Develop a Shredded Exec Mindset. Now let's get to the tips you need to make part of your daily routine. Regarding lifestyle, nutrition, supplements, hydration, and other things.

Step #1. Eat right at night.

Want to know what most people do wrong that leads to poor sleep? They eat a big, high-carb meal at night. Don't eat a high-carb meal before bed. Not because it's going to make you fat, (which it will if you eat trash or eat too many calories), but because of the effects it has on your hormones. If you eat high-carb meal before bed, you are going to spike blood sugar, which triggers insulin (fat storage hormone) that will also blunt the release of a really awesome hormone called Human Growth Hormone. HGH is a muscle builder and fat burner. We want HGH at night. Insulin (storage hormone) also blunts fat burning.

Eating a high carb meal also messes up other hormonal systems, which can prevent you from falling into REM sleep and sleeping fully. If you have terrible sleep will also lead to waking up with higher cortisol levels, which make you craving more carbs, feeling lethargic and lacking energy all day. So the last meal of your day to promote the proper release of the best balance of hormones would simply be protein, veggies, and good fats. This will keep your blood sugar in check, promote the release of all the good hormones and you will sleep deeply and wake up like a champ.

Step #2. Get your magnesium.

Want to know a simple trick that takes seconds that can make you sleep like a BABY? Take a high-quality magnesium supplement about 30-60 minutes before bed. In case you don't know, magnesium is responsible for over 350 chemical reactions on the body, and SLEEP is one of them. Most people are extremely deficient due to their poor nutrition and lifestyles. Even if you do eat healthy, I promise you are still deficient. So supplement it!

Most supplements on the market are synthetic crap. You need a high-quality magnesium supplement for this trick to work. The ONLY brand I recommend is called Mega Food. You can find it at some grocery stores like Sprouts, Mothers, and if you google it, you can buy it online by just searching for the keywords: "Mega Food Magnesium."

Take four to six pills every night before bed. Just keep the bottle on your nightstand so you remember daily. You will quickly see how incredible this one trick will make you feel when you wake up in the morning. This mineral is seriously magic; you will sleep and dream vividly like a champ. You may wake up going "WTF that was a crazy dream?!!" I do that often and that's a comment I also hear from clients.

Magnesium is also responsible for energy production and muscle contractions, so like I said it is the magic mineral that will not only improve your sleep, it will give you more energy and improve workout effectiveness.

Step #3. Plan for success.

Want to know one of the key things that almost ALL very successful high achievers do at night? They plan their to-do list each night for the next day. Each night, along with writing down your daily goals, plan your top three to five things you need to do for the next day. What this does is it organizes your thoughts, makes you focused, and programs your mind for the next day. Your brain will be processing this information while you sleep and you will wake up focused! You may even get a brilliant idea while you're asleep, so keep your notes nearby to write it down if you wake up. This is common.

Step #4. Drown the fatigue.

Want to know the real reason why you wake up feeling like crap daily? Dehydration. You haven't had any fluids in at least six to eight hours and you've been losing them every second. When you wake up you're dry like a desert, which slows down ALL of your bodily systems, especially ENERGY production. One of the tricks to waking up refreshed is to make sure you drank an adequate amount each day and before bed. Hydrate as soon as your alarm goes off. You should be consuming 1.5 - 3 gallons of water per day if you want to look and feel like a fuvking champ daily.

Most of you don't even get near this, which is why you feel like crap daily. Then you guzzle coffee to compensate, when all you needed was WATER. So drink adequate water daily, then keep a protein shaker cup, or glass next to your bed already filled with water and a teaspoon of Himalayan or sea salt. As soon as your alarm goes off, sit up, put your feet on the floor, and DOWN that water.

Step #5. Stand up to welcome the day!

As soon as that water is down, stand up and walk to your bathroom, splash water on your face, and start brushing your teeth. Within a few minutes, the salt water will hit your system and you will start to feel energized. Until then, FORCE it. Snooze is not allowed. Snooze is for people who are broke. If you want to be a success, snooze is NEVER an option.

What did I just say? Snoozing is NOT an option. Alarm beeps, man the fuvk up and follow the first 5 steps.

Step #6. Habit.

How long does it take to create a habit? Twenty-one days? Thirty days? This is a controversial topic depending on your source, but with my research on the latest findings, science has proven it takes up to 66 days on average to ingrain a habit. Some sooner, some much longer. To create this habit you need to commit to waking up EVERY single day until it becomes a habit.

Yes, this includes weekends. Even if you only get up on the weekend for an hour, then go back and take a nap, DO IT. Get up, go do some work, write down your goals, do something productive, get up to establish consistency and ingrain the habit. Then if you're still tired, go take a little nap.

We are communicating to your subconscious that "You wake up early. You are a morning person. You do what you intend to do. This is who you are." Once you ingrain this habit, it's EASY to wake up early. You start to enjoy it, enjoy how much more you get done, enjoy having so much more time to spend with your family because you didn't have to work or train so late.

There you have it. Those are the six steps how to become a morning person. Do those DAILY and create the habit.

Now once you are up, what do you do? It's simple, really. The most successful people do a few things when they wake up which is why they are successful.

1. Create positive emotion in the morning.

How do we create a positive emotions? Gratitude, along with setting goals and to-do lists. The best way to start your day off on a positive note is by writing down the top three to five things you are grateful for each morning. It's not successful people that are happy, its happy people that become successful. By starting your day off focusing on what you love, appreciate and are thankful for, you start your day with positive emotions and your mind will be giving off these vibes and focused on looking for more positive things.

Gratitude is the precursor to happiness, and the root of everything you want is HAPPINESS. Being happy is a choice, and you can choose to have it NOW and it begins with starting your day off with your top three to five things you're grateful for. So put it on paper. Then write down your goals. There is so much power in seeing your goals in writing.

"Those who write their goals down are 1000% more successful than those who do not."
- Brian Tracy.

Studies have proven time and again that those who put their goals in writing achieve a TREMENDOUS amount more than people who do not, so establish this habit daily. This also prepares your mind, makes you focused on achieving them. Then review the top three to-do's for the day. This is a simple but powerful thing that almost every single high-achieving CEO or entrepreneur does. So DO IT!

2. Get In the gym.

One of the best ways to make your training a habit is to get it done first thing in the morning. Most people are too tired to go to the gym after work, which leads to them using the old, "I'm tired, I'll go tomorrow" excuse, which we all know leads to YEARS of missed workouts. So to avoid this and start making consistent progress, start scheduling your workouts FIRST thing in the morning. You will get your endorphin high, get your energy levels up, and have your workout completed your workout for the day.

You don't have to spend an hour in the gym, but you do need to work out EVERY day. Even if you are pressed for time, that day, just go in to bust out a quick 15 to 30-minute workout to ingrain this habit. Whatever it takes, get your ass in the gym seven days a week. If you're super beat up and sore, so what? Take your ass to the gym and stretch, do the sauna, and roll out muscles. This sends a message to your subconscious that this is who you are and what you do. Form this habit.

2. Tackle the most important task.

After training, get to work! Each morning you have the silence to focus, no distractions, no kids bugging, no spouse talking to you, just you and the ability to tackle the day's most important task. You have the endorphin high from your workout to help you tackle that one task that I know you've procrastinated on doing. Tackling that big one this sets you up for success the rest of the day. So each morning after training, focus on tackling the ONE thing that is going to move your business or finances forward.

4. Personal development.

If you're successful, you already know this but I will reiterate it: the only way you are going to achieve GREATNESS is by improving YOURSELF. You must read and listen to personal development books DAILY. The top earning CEOs read over 60 books a YEAR, while the average person reads less than one. These same CEOs earn 319 times more than the average person. Connect the dots. These high achievers constantly devour information and apply it to their selves, businesses, lives and this is WHY they are high achievers.

Millionaires, top earning CEOs, and successful entrepreneurs aren't wasting their time watching *"The Voice"* or *"American Idol."* Instead, they watch their businesses and bank accounts grow because they constantly put in the work on their personal growth.

If you have time to watch TV, you have time to read or train. If you have time to listen to music, you have time to learn. Get the Audible.com app on your smartphone so you can listen to audiobooks while driving, cooking, or down time. Successful people don't piss away their time like average people do.

Average people watch five hours of TV a day – statistically they spend 37 hours a week invested in useless entertainment. That's a full-time job worth of time invested on NOTHING. This same average person in America is also fat, broke, and struggles financially. According to the Social Security Administration, 95% of Americans struggle financially – another connect the dots moment.

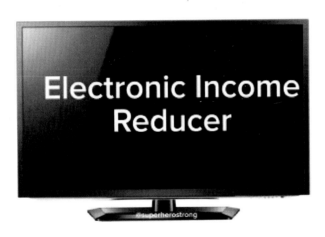

This is why the TV is called the "Electronic Income Reducer". It is proven that the more TV you watch, the less you earn.

"To earn more, you must first LEARN more."
–Brian Tracy

To become part of that elite top 1 to 5%, you have to do what they do, and that's continually learning and improving. That includes rereading this book and learning more about nutrition.

Continue this by reading business, personal development books, and other topics to enrich your mind.

Improve yourself and you improve your life. As you improve, everything in your life will as well. Turn your drive time into a university on wheels. Listen to audiobooks while commuting EVERY day. Watch how much more awesome you become in the office and how much more successful you become.

So there you go, six tips on how to become a morning person and four tips on what to do when you wake up. I personally follow all of them myself and I wake at 4:00 a.m. seven days a week. My life today is phenomenal, and the best is yet to come! I'm still on my way up!

I threw in some extra tips here because as I said in the beginning, not only do I want you shredded, I want you WEALTHY! Follow these rules. Improve yourself and all of these small daily actions will compound to greatness and success over time. To live like the shredded and successful do, you have to DO what the shredded and successful do.

Review:

1. What should you NOT eat before bed?
2. What should you eat as your last meal?
3. How many magnesium tablets should you take before bed?
4. What brand? Why only that brand?
5. Along with writing your goals each night, what else should you do in writing?
6. What's the real reason you are fatigued each morning? What is the first thing you need to do as soon as alarm goes off?
7. What goes in your water?

8. As soon as you're done drinking water, what are the next few steps?
9. How many days does it take to really ingrain a habit?
10. How many days a week should you wake up early to develop a habit?
11. What four things do you need to do upon waking?

[6]

Shredded Executive Nutrition 101

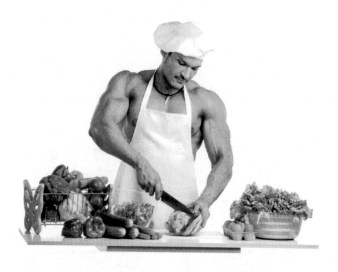

Would you like to know why Americans are so sick and so fat? Want to know why people cannot control their eating behaviors? How about why people are so lazy, lethargic, and rarely hit the gym? Why when you eat those tasty foods, you can't stop? Want to know why it is that we have an obesity and chronic disease epidemic?

The biggest mistake in the history of nutrition

The "war" on saturated fat which was launched in 1977, is the biggest mistake in the history of nutrition. People reduced their intake of animal fat and cholesterol, because flawed studies led us to believe that it was the fats causing heart disease.

I could write an entire book on this topic alone but I'll spare you the time. Just know that over 70+ studies have conclusively shown that neither saturated fat nor dietary cholesterol causes harm in humans. Saturated fat has NOTHING to do with heart disease, as matter of fact, countries with the highest intake of saturated fats have LOWER incidents of heart disease deaths.

This low-fat era that started in 1977 is what actually sparked our obesity epidemic, it wasn't the fats in foods causing our heart disease issue back then. Instead, it was the high-carb, highly processed food diets and poor lifestyles of Americans. The reason this was the biggest mistake in history is because the launch of the low-fat era, prompted food companies started taking the fats out of foods. They started making "fat-free, low-fat, reduced fat options". When you take fats out of foods, they taste like cardboard, so guess what they added IN to make them more palatable?

I'm sure you guessed it: SUGAR!

BOOM! This began the launch of our obesity epidemic that is now leading to the astronomical rates of obese, overweight, and high body fat Americans. It has led to the insane epidemic of various chronic disease.

Although numerous studies have proven that a high-fat diet is actually HEALTHIER than a low-fat diet, studies prove high-fat diets are more effective for fat loss and make you look good and feel great, but the average person is not aware of this yet. The typical medical community is still preaching low-fat because they are not up to speed on the latest nutritional science, nor are they adequately trained in nutrition. They are outdated, and typically 8 - 10 years behind the curve.

We can discuss this topic for DAYS on end, so to save you the time, understand the low-fat era has since been DEBUNKED. It has been proven over and over that there is NO correlation between saturated fat and heart disease, nor cholesterol in food leading to plaque in arteries.

So if you hear anyone, a doctor, friend, or anyone preaching low fat, RUN! They are outdated fools. I don't care how shredded they are or the title they carry. They obviously haven't been keeping up to date with science and pursuing low-fat diet will lead to health issues, hormone issues, issues with bodily functions, and set you up for binging.

Just know, the fats are NOT going to give you high cholesterol and they are not going to clog your arteries. As matter of fact, it is quite the opposite. Sugar is what causes heart attacks. Processed foods that spike blood sugar are what damages arteries. Having high blood sugar is like taking sandpaper to your arteries. Science has proven it, and it's time the world catches up with science.

Fats are excellent for your health, energy, nutrient absorption, and helping you to get shredded. Examples of good fat sources are: nuts, seeds, avocado, natural peanut butter, grass-fed butter, coconut oil, and animal fats from healthy animals.

When we get to the nutrition portion of this book, I will give you examples of an ideal healthy, quality nutrition plan that is full of good fats, good carbs, and good proteins. This plan is going to make you LOOK incredible, feel incredible, and have vibrant health.

Just know that fat is your FRIEND. Sugar is your nemesis.

Sugar is a drug that comes in many forms

"Sugar is eight times more addictive than cocaine."
-Dr. Mark Hyman

This includes all processed foods(bread, pasta, cereal) because they are converted to sugar as soon as you ingest them. Sugar and processed foods are HIGHLY addictive and the number one reason why YOU are carrying that excess layer of chub over your abs.

Sugar is also the number one reason why almost 70% of Americans are obese, overweight, and sick. I believe that this number is more like 95%. Because the current standards are based off of BMI(height, weight), I bet that if we did actual body fat tests on every American, we would find our obesity/overweight epidemic is more like 95%. It's terrible and worse than you can even imagine. In my years of training, doing very rigorous body fat skin fold testing, this is what I have found to be true. The average person is fatter than they think, they are fatter than the doctors think, and fatter than they look.

Average looking people carrying 20, 30, or over 50 excess pounds of body fat. They may not be heavy on the scale but have very low levels of lean body mass and high levels of body fat. Today the average height and weight of a man in America today is 5'9", around 195 pounds, with almost a 40-inch waist. A 40-inch waist! That's insane!

A 5'9" man should be around 170 pounds, well-developed, and shredded up to 185 pounds (if he's jacked), with a 28 to 30-inch waist average.

An average 5'9" man weighing 195 pounds is easily carrying a good 40+ EXCESS lbs. of pure body fat. So even though he's only 10 to 25 pounds heavier than what his ideal weight should be on the scale, the amount of muscle he has is low and his body fat is very high.

For example, let's take Shredded Exec Mike and Average Exec Joe:

- Mike is 170 lbs. with 5% body fat.
- Joe is 195 lbs. with 25% body fat. (This is very common.)
- Mike at 5% body fat has 161.5 lbs. of lean body mass (bones, organs, and muscle) on his frame, and is only carrying 8.5 lbs. of body fat. Very low body fat means excellent condition.
- Joe at 25% body fat on the other hand, has 146 lbs. of lean body mass on his frame, and he is carrying almost 49 lbs. of fat.

The scale only tells part of the story. Body fat testing tells it all. So even though there is only a 25 pound scale weight difference between the two (Joe is 195 – Mike is 170), there is over a 40 pound difference between how much fat they are carrying. The difference between how they look is VASTLY different. Mike is shredded; you can see the striations, lines, and contours of all his muscles, shredded abs, and is turning heads everywhere he goes. Joe, well Joe is just FAT, average, and no one even notices him or looks twice – because he looks average. At 25% body fat, Joe is actually clinically obese. He looks average, but his body fat is so high that he's technically obese.

This is why the system we use in America to determine one's health is a little flawed. It's based off of height and weight (BMI), which is not an accurate assessment of one's health or composition. Hell, according to my BMI, I'm actually considered overweight because I'm short, even though I'm lean, well developed, and in phenomenal health. See, height and weight doesn't paint the whole picture.

So why is Joe and everyone so fat?

Because Americans are drug addicts. Their top two drugs of choice are sugar and flour (bread, pasta, pizza, cake, cookies, cereal, soda, sports drinks, etc.). In case you're not aware, these are ALL sugar. Flour converts to sugar as soon as you consume it and science has proven these sugars are eight times more addictive than cocaine. EIGHT TIMES! The average American eats around 150 lbs. of sugar per year and around 150 lbs. of flour per year. Wow! That's almost a pound a day of sugar-like foods.

What makes these so addictive?

These are addictive because they trigger dopamine. One bite or sip leads to a dopamine high (that lights up the pleasure centers of your brain like a Christmas tree), like illegal drugs do. You see, it's not that the "taste" of these foods that you love. Rather, it's that these foods make you "FEEL" good from the dopamine high. It is this high that is the REAL reason you crave those foods, the real reason why you drool when you think about pizza, donuts, ice cream, bread, pasta, and restaurant foods.

It's the HIGH, the feeling you're chasing, that is the real reason why one bite usually leads to uncontrollable overeating. You probably even just got cravings from me just mentioning those foods. This is exactly my point, that's how powerful this addiction is. Just like a drug addict is always chasing the next hit to keep his high going, people keep chasing the high once they taste foods that light up their reward centers of their brain.

This is also one of the reasons you have failed over and over to eat a healthy, whole food diet. You do good for a couple days or weeks, then go to a dinner or social setting and have a bite of something processed, like pizza, cake, or from something you see or smell – and BAM! You're on a binge and back off the wagon. Because you reignited the addiction, the cravings continue for up to 72 hours later or longer, which is why most people end up bingeing for days. This is why for most people – 99.99% of you – cannot just have one bite or one serving, because one taste leads to surge of dopamine and you binge to keep the high going. For days, weeks, and months.

Why is this so common?

Because foods companies spend millions of dollars creating the right ratio of sugar, salt, and fat to create what they call the "bliss" level so they sell more products. These foods are literally DESIGNED to be addictive.

Sugar is in almost EVERYTHING. Food companies add it in processed foods because they know it will create a raving fan, an addict, who will keep purchasing their products and increase their profits. Restaurants have it in their ingredients of your favorite dishes, along with lots of other ingredients that are highly stimulating, highly addictive, and truly terrible for your health and waistline. This is why you always go to your favorite restaurants to eat your favorite dish. The food addiction called and you answered.

Sugar is everywhere. It's in bread, pasta, spaghetti sauce, chips, coffee creamers, tortillas, protein powders, protein bars, and in almost ALL foods created by man. For example, the typical spaghetti sauce has more added sugar than a few Oreo cookies. Didn't know that, huh? It comes in many forms, with many different names. So even though a product may be organic, claim "no sugar," it could have a form of sugar in it. It's just called something like "evaporated cane juice/syrup, agave, or fructose," just to name a few. These are not technically "sugar," the refined added sugar, but still a form of sugar that can have a similar surge in blood sugar levels. They also trigger dopamine, which leads to more cravings, which leads to more over consuming.

Sugar equals cravings for more sugar. This includes artificial sweeteners. Yes, this includes calorie-free, Stevia, and all of it. There is no free lunch. Sweet makes you crave more sweets and more carbs. Period.

It's a vicious cycle.

Along with the cravings, sugar also triggers insulin, which is a fat-storing hormone. When you consume carbs of any sort, the body releases a hormone called insulin to shuttle the blood sugar to cells. When you consume sugar, you're going to spike blood sugar rapidly. Insulin swoops in to pull that blood sugar down because it is toxic to be that high.

But what happens is insulin usually overcompensates and pulls your blood sugar down too low. This is the crash. This leaves you fatigued, wanting a nap, and craving more carbs or sugar. When your blood sugar and insulin spikes like that, it makes your body want to store fat. Whatever carbs are not burned immediately, and your muscles are full of glycogen (stored carbs), all excess calories get stored as fat.

This is why if you start with the bread or chips at a restaurant, this spikes blood sugar, triggers dopamine, ignites food addiction, and you always end up eating a lot more than you wanted to. Add in liquid sugar (soda, alcohol, sweeteners in tea), and your consumption is off the charts. You binge eat, over-consume, and keep eating even though you're full, store fat, wake up in the morning, and look in the mirror with regret and cravings. Sound familiar? I know it does.

> *"You are eating yourself to death. Digging your grave with your teeth."*
> *–Daymond Sewall*

What's worse than being fat?

Being diseased and unhealthy. The top killers each year are not the murderers, not terrorists, and not car accidents. They are chronic diseases, diseases that are scientifically PROVEN to be caused by DIET and lifestyle. Terrible nutrition, poor lifestyles, and nutrient deficiencies lead to the body breaking. Every year, about 600,000 Americans die from heart disease and every year, 720,000 have heart attacks. Every year, 1,665,540 new cancer cases are diagnosed and 585,720 people die from cancer. There are 29 million Americans with diabetes, another 86 million with pre-diabetes. Each year, over 1.5 million Americans die annually from these chronic diseases that are DIET and LIFESTYLE related conditions.

Diseases that are created by our own doing and are preventable. Yes, you heard that right. Science has proven that these are DIET and LIFESTYLE related diseases. Now I'm not going to go in detail in this book about disease, but know heart disease, most cancers, Type 2 diabetes, stroke, and Alzheimer's, are the leading killers. ALL of them preventable diseases. REALLY? Yes, really! This is scientifically proven. Do your homework.

These diseases are running rampant because Americans LIVE off processed foods, which are destroying their health, jacking up their hormones, depleting their nutrients, and killing them slowly. Americans are literally eating themselves to death.

This is why everyone is so fat, why we have an obesity epidemic, and why everyone is sick. We have all lost loved ones to these diseases. What could have happened if they had the knowledge that we have today?

How would our lives be if we still had them with us? I too have lost many, many family members to these diseases. This is why I am so passionate about educating YOU about these things, so YOU don't become a statistic and YOU create a ripple effect of change to those around you.

Change begins NOW.

It starts with food

So now that you know why you have excess body fat, you know why you have cravings, you know why you have pain, and you know why your health may be suffering, what are you doing to do about it? How do you gain control over an addiction so you gain control over your health, your mind, your body and your results?

How does someone get rid an addiction? Whether its alcohol or crack, how do they eliminate a substance abuse issue? Kick the habit! Right or right?

They go cold turkey. This is an addiction – worse than a drug addiction. So just like a drug addiction, you have to kick the habit cold turkey. There is no weaning off and no doing it slowly. If you had the kind of discipline to just have a little, you'd be shredded right now. You're not shredded yet, so that says you DON'T have that kind of discipline. To gain control over your mind and body, you need to detox from the sugar addiction.

How to kick the habit

That means starting RIGHT now, cut out ALL processed foods. Bread, pasta, cereals, bagels, pizza, soda, coffee creamers, fat free products(sugar bombs), donuts, cake and any other food that was made by man. You will have withdrawals, you will detox, you will have cravings, and you will be a mess for a few days.

Get past Day 3

You will be a mess, but just remember, it's only temporary. For most of you, all you have to do is get past Day 3. Day 3 for most people is the peak of the cravings, withdrawals, and this is the day you will probably want to choke someone or cry. You may experience headaches, shaking, sweats, achy muscles, along with the cravings and moodiness. This is how powerful this drug is. Until now, you had no idea how bad your problem was. The good news is for most people by Days 4 and 5, you'll feel better and better each day.

Day 7: "OMG, I feel so good!"

If you did it right, cut out ALL manmade foods, and kicked the sugar addiction, by Day 7 you will feel AWESOME! The most common response I hear from clients is usually, "OMG! I feel so good. Why didn't I do this sooner?!"

Most people don't realize just how shitty they have been feeling until they experience what it's like to feel GOOD. Most people walk around fatigued, tired, weak, with brain fog, feeling terrible all day. But because terrible is all they know, its normal to them. However, when your body is healthy, when your hormones are in check and when you're giving the body the nutrition and nutrients it truly wants, you feel AMAZING. Your energy levels SOAR, your productivity increases, your workouts are awesome, you are more happy, you feel great, and above all, you burn fat and get shredded!

So kick the habit, pull your panties up, and hold on tight to get past the peak of Day 3.

This includes protein shakes, protein bars, and processed meats. All of these have added sugars/sweeteners. Cut those too.

So what are you allowed to eat?

Good question. I have made the rule of nutrition very simple to follow: **EAT REAL FOOD.**

What is REAL food?

"If it came directly from a plant, or it had a mom, this is real food. EAT IT."

–Daymond Sewall

These are one-ingredient foods. These are foods made by nature, came directly from a plant, or had a mom. When it comes to food, just ask yourself this question "Did it come DIRECTLY from a plant? Did it have a mom?" If so, then YES, it's approved.

If it had to be made by man, in a factory, or has a list of ingredients, it means its processed junk and it's NOT approved. EVER. Just think of them as a poison and the side effect is body fat and disease. Now let's talk about real food.

So what comes from a plant?

VEGGIES (of all colors), nuts, seeds, fruit, etc. Just an FYI: fruit is a carb and it is NOT a free food. Just because it's healthy doesn't mean it won't make you fat. Fruit is a natural sugar and overeaten can make you fat, like other forms of sugar. Fruit has LIMITS. As does quinoa, oats, beans, brown rice and other high-carb sources. We will discuss that later.

Most nuts and seeds are considered good fats. Almonds, macadamia, cashews, and sunflower are examples of nuts and seeds that are good fat sources.

So what foods come from a mom?

Chicken, beef, pork, turkey, fish, eggs, etc. These are also your protein sources. Some of these protein sources will have a lot of fats in them as well. This is good, because you NEED fats. Fats are crucial to your health, hormones (testosterone, growth hormone), cellular function, metabolism, and health.

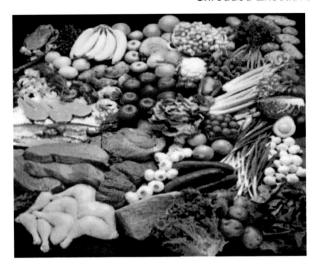

PVF: Always eat Protein and Veggies First!

The staple for every single one of your meals is ALWAYS protein and veggies. Some meals will have more carbs or fats added to them, but the staple for ALL meals is **PVF.** So know that every meal, every day, you are going to be eating protein and veggies first before you eat anything. This one thing is what will set you up for optimal health, the best hormonal balance, keep you blood sugar in check, energy levels high, provide best environment for recovery, and help you get SHREDDED!

When we get to the meal plan section, you will see what I mean. For now, starting right now, eat protein and veggies every meal. As you read further, you will see example nutrition plans of what to eat and how to eat, but for now just eat protein and veggies.

So what is the staple for every meal?

PVF! Simple, right? Good. Now let's talk about a quick little BELIEF to establish that will help you with this discipline.

Improve your belief system

"What you believe is what you experience."
-Unknown

Want to learn a simple mindset hack that will help you create good nutritional habits? Want to know an easy belief to instill that will help you keep your diet on point?

A simple hack to put into your belief system is "I don't eat that." This refers to processed foods, foods that contain sugar/flour, or foods that could contain these ingredients. If you have the belief that you just don't eat those types of foods, then you have no problem avoiding them. So instead of feeling like "I can't eat that," which may just make you want to eat it more, by programming the belief "I don't eat that," it's not even an option. This is one of my personal beliefs and hacks. This is one of the beliefs that I teach my clients to develop as well.

Everyone knows that everywhere I go, "I just don't eat that." If I go places and there is a dish that someone made, or at restaurants, if it looks like it could even possibly have flour or sugar in ingredients, I won't touch it. I'm always first to ask "What's in it? What's it made with?" I have NO problem turning things down or avoiding certain foods.

Why? Because truly the EASY way of getting shredded and staying shredded is eating only REAL food. Think about it: I don't have to deal with cravings. I don't have to worry about the risk igniting the food addiction and overeating. I won't have to deal with cravings for DAYS after. I also don't want to risk getting an injury in training from the inflammation these foods cause.

So what is the belief you want to program?

"I don't eat that!"

Want to know how I train year-round?

Want to know one of my secrets of how I train year round and rarely take a day off? (As of writing this book the only day I have taken off was the birth of my son ABS. I was on a 320 day streak before that)

The other reason why you want to eliminate these foods and instill the belief "I don't eat that" is because they are highly damaging to your gut health, which leads to systemic inflammation. Systemic inflammation is a nasty side effect of eating processed foods which creates joint and muscle pain in almost EVERYONE.

Processed foods = Pain

The inflammation tightens up muscles, flares up knotted tissues, and flares up old injuries that cause pain. One bite of those foods can mean a pulled muscle, achy joints, random muscle pain, back pain, knee pain, or shoulder pain for up to 7-14 days AFTER you eat it.

If you are in pain, are you going to be able to train hard to get shredded? Are you going to be able to lift as heavy as you need to produce results? If your back hurts, can you squat, deadlift, row, or even pickup weights to train other body parts? No, no, and no. This inflammation would impede your ability to train effectively and slow down your intensity, which slows your results. It's NOT worth it!

If you have chronic pain now or have a joint or muscle issue that you're currently working around, now you know why. Its not because you are old, its because you are inflamed. Cut these foods and watch the pain disappear and how awesome you feel in about two weeks.

So if you know that processed foods or food containing sugar, flour, or manmade products are highly inflammatory and will slow down your progress, what are you going to COMMIT to doing so you can get shredded as fast as possible? Avoid them at all costs! Yes or yes? Good.

The reason I am able to train nonstop year round is because I keep my diet clean ALL year. No processed food, no pain. No pain, no missed sessions. My diet is full of nutritious foods which speed recovery and keep my body healthy and strong.

A whole food diet is the secret. **EAT REAL FOOD.**

What do I consider real food? Remember, nutrition simplified in one sentence: "If it came directly from a plant, or it came directly from an animal, you CAN EAT it." So when it comes to food if you're ever in doubt ask yourself, "Did this come directly from a plant? Did this come from an animal?" If yes, its approved. If no, it's forbidden. If it was processed or made by man, it does not belong in your body.

Set up your kitchen for success

What does this mean? One of the first steps to setting yourself up for success is eliminating the temptations. This means set your home up for your success to get shredded.

Go through you kitchen and toss out ALL foods that came packaged, boxed, and all items that were made by man. These foods include bread, pasta, cereal, sweeteners, soda, diet soda, sports drinks, fruit juices, candy, ice cream, tortillas, yogurts, cheese (inflammatory for most people), and yes, this includes ALL wheat products. Throw them out. Yes, that means waste the food. But remember, this is not food. These are drugs, toxins, double chins, and muffin tops in a package. Throw it away. It's not real food.

REAL food doesn't cause inflammation. REAL food delivers nutrition, vitamins, minerals, and healthy protein, carbs, fats to your muscles. EAT REAL FOOD. So go through your cabinets, through your fridge, and throw away ALL processed manmade foods.

Why do you think this is such an important step? Because addiction is POWERFUL. If it is in your home, you WILL crave it. You will be tempted. One bad day, one stressful day, and you'll be inhaling bon-bons and watch *"The Notebook"* like a little bitch.

So get the shit out of your house now! Go! DO IT NOW! DTFW!

What belongs in your kitchen?

Now that your kitchen is cleaned up, what foods should you keep in it? Fill your fridge and kitchen with REAL food, veggies of all colors, fruit, nuts, seeds, healthy animal proteins (grass-fed, organic, and wild caught). These are REAL foods. These are the foods our bodies are designed to eat. These are the foods that provide the proper macros (protein, carbs, fats) and micros (vitamins and minerals) that our bodies need to function optimally. These are the foods that are going to make you look incredible, have vibrant health, tons of energy and make you Feel AMAZING. These foods will not trigger cravings, will not cause inflammation, and they help you keep your calorie intake in check.

If you don't have cravings, can account for every calorie, and can train like a beast all week, what's going to happen? You're going to get fuvking shredded! Yes or yes?!

Okay, we talked about the basics about food, so I'm sure you're wondering what you can drink.

What can I drink?

WATER should be the primary thing you drink all day. No soda, diet sodas, sports drinks, coconut water, vitamin waters – NONE of that. Why? Because these are packed with sugar and/or artificial sweeteners. Drink WATER instead.

There are a couple things you can drink: coffee and tea. But these DO NOT count as your water intake. You still need to drink the recommended water intake as well.

Coffee

If you drink coffee, drink it black or with 28g of grass-fed butter blended in it (it's amazing), or with coconut oil blended in it. That's the ONLY thing you are allowed to put in your coffee. Why? Because I know you want to put creamers, what do you think creamers are? Sugar and sweeteners, which are forbidden. Either drink it like I suggested or not at all.

If you drink tea, drink it plain. If you cannot drink these like this, then you really don't like them. It was the sugar or artificial sweetener you were after all these years. Your number one fluid you should be consuming lots of is PURE water.

Shredder Nutrition

We have discussed the foods to avoid, and the only foods you should be eating. Now it's time to talk a little bit of science so you understand what food really is. The way we do things is very simple but its strategic and pure science. I am going to keep it short and just give you the nuts and bolts.

Macros

"The key to getting shredded is to be on point with your macros seven days a week."
- Daymond Sewall

WTF are macros?

I get this question a lot, especially on social media. I'm sure you have heard this term before and I have mentioned it a few times in the previous chapters. But just in case you still aren't sure what these are, macros is short for *macronutrients*. Macros are your protein, carbs and fats measured in grams. We talk a lot about calories but know not all calories are the same, different macros have different metabolic pathways and release different hormones. They have different effects on energy, appetite, fat burning, muscle building and maintenance and your testosterone/growth hormone levels.

So although calories are the most important aspect, you MUST get an appropriate amount of protein and fats in your diet to maintain, develop muscle, and get shredded. Notice I didn't mention carbs? That's because carbs are the ONLY macro we can live without. The primary purpose of carbs is for energy, but because protein and fats can be converted to energy, we can literally live without carbs. With that said, carbs cannot do what fats and proteins do. Carbs cannot provide the building blocks for muscle, cellular development, or hormones which are why carbs are the least important. This is why when it comes to manipulation of the diet to achieve a specific caloric intake, it's the carbs that get either cut to create a calorie deficit or increased to refeed. This is why we will be carb cycling.

Don't worry if you don't know anything about what I just said regarding deficit, refeed, and carb cycling, because I will explain in a moment. For now, just pay attention. The more you know and understand WHY you are doing things, the more you will do things the right way. Just know when I say macros, I'm referring to your protein, carbs and fat.

Just an FYI: each gram of carbs is four calories, each gram of protein is four calories, each gram of fat is nine calories. You will be eating a specific macro ratio you will achieve your desired calorie intake. For instance, a diet that consists of 90 g carbs, 240 g protein, 120 g fats is 2,400 calories. We focus on macros to achieve a specific calorie intake to create a fat burning environment, but also to give your body the raw materials it needs to develop muscles, maintain muscles, develop hormones, and keep your blood sugar levels in check. Creating the correct calorie intake by hitting your macros daily is KEY to getting shredded.

Not all calories are created equal

A calorie is simply a unit of energy that the human body uses to perform the basic functions of life. The amount of calories your body will need is truly dependent on your build (amount of muscle, height, weight, etc.) and the activity you do on a daily basis. "A calorie is a calorie" when its measured in a LAB. But the human body is a highly complex biochemical system with elaborate processes to regulate your energy balance. Different foods go through different pathways, some of which are inefficient and some of those calories are lost due to digestion.

Even more important is the fact that different macros have a direct effect on the hormones and brain centers that control hunger and your behaviors. This is why a calorie is NOT just a calorie. Although calories are the number one determining factor of fat burning or fat storing, they are NOT created equal. Like I just said, protein and carbs both contain four calories each, while fats contain nine calories each. However, they all have different metabolic and hormonal responses in the body.

For example, 750 calories of soda (sugar/carbs) will have a completely different effect than 750 calories from broccoli (carbs). Both are the same amount of calories, but they will all have a different response on your hormones and metabolism. Seven hundred and fifty calories of soda will spike your blood sugar, trigger a burst of insulin (fat storing hormone), make you have a blood sugar crash about an hour later, leaving you fatigued wanting a nap, only to crave more carbs/sugar to bring your blood sugar back up. This eventually leads to your overconsumption and leads to you getting fatter.

Seven hundred and fifty calories from broccoli, which is also a carb, will make you FULL for the rest of the day! I dare you to try and eat 750 calories from broccoli. You will not have a blood sugar spike and it stabilizes your blood sugar. It is full of fiber, which is a crucial element of health and keeping your digestion in check so it can absorb nutrients optimally. It has micronutrients (vitamins and minerals) which are the raw materials your body needs for health and to perform its best. This vegetable will naturally make you eat less, which means more fat burning for you and you getting shredded.

Seven hundred and fifty calories from protein will have a completely metabolic and hormonal response. Protein kills appetite, which also makes you eat fewer calories, which means more DEFICIT and fat loss for you. Studies have also shown that high-protein diets have a metabolic advantage and boost metabolism by up to 100 calories per day. Protein does not spike blood sugar, will keep you fuller, and will help you control your food intake. It will provide consistent energy and the building blocks your body needs for every cell in your body.

So even though the calories are the same and will burn equally in a lab environment, the macros you eat to achieve your designated calorie intake have different effects on hunger, hormones, energy expenditure, and the brain regions that control food intake. All of these ultimately affect your performance, bodily functions, health and results.

Macro categories

Most people are unaware of which foods are which, and thanks to the vegan community, they have confused the hell out of people. I'm going to give you a quick lesson on what is considered a protein, a carb, and a fat.

Proteins

What foods do you think are proteins? This one is an easy one, this is primarily our animal sources. ALL foods that came from a "mom" are considered our proteins. This includes eggs, chicken, fish, beef, pork, turkey, etc.

Yes, there are some proteins in veggies, grains and fruit too, but it's very, very small. Where some people get confused is they think quinoa, oats, beans, and nuts are proteins. Wrong. Thank you vegans, you just confused an already confused society. Just an FYI, quinoa, beans, and oats are three to five times HIGHER in carbs than they are protein.

For example, one cup of cooked quinoa has 39 grams of carbs and only eight grams protein. That means it has over four times MORE carbs than protein. See, it's a CARB source, not a protein source. Get it right, vegans!

Some protein sources you will eat have higher fat content, so when eating these types, you won't need to add additional fats to those meals. For example, Atlantic Salmon, grass-fed ground beef, and chicken thighs have a good amount of fats in them. As you learn more about food, which you will with experience, you will see what I mean. With that said, although we do need fats, they are very calorie-dense, so be very accurate with your intake daily.

Protein's role

What is protein and what is it used for? By definition, it is organic compounds of large molecules composed of chains of amino acids. The body breaks down protein into specific amino acids and then selectively put together for different uses. These new proteins formed in the body are what make up most of the solid matter in the body. Solid matter like skin, eyes, hair, nails, cartilage, blood, heart, intestines, bones and of course, MUSCLE. It is also needed to make some enzymes, hormones, and other body chemicals.

The body needs a relatively large amount of it daily. But unlike fat and carbs, the body does not store excess protein, so it does not have a reservoir to draw from when it needs a new supply. It must be supplied by the diet daily. Protein is one of the key macros to you developing a shredded physique. It is required for the development and maintenance of muscle. It is the key building block for muscle repair from workouts. I'm sure you know that, but it also has many other purposes you may not know:

- Adequate protein intake also naturally improves your body composition by eliminating hunger, keeping you fuller, which means natural calorie reduction(deficit) and lower body fat levels.
- Protein improves strength, bone density, and your sleep.
- Protein at around 25-30% or more of your daily calorie intake has also been shown to boost metabolism by up to 100 calories per day.
- Protein eaten every meal also keeps your blood sugar more stable, which is a key component of melting fat. Because it slows the digestion of any carbs eaten, your blood sugar rises slowly, and will fall slowly, meaning good clean energy for you. No blood sugar spiking and crashing which is what most people have all day from the sugar/flour/processed foods most people eat.

But when it comes to you and your diet, the primary reasons we have the rule PVF (protein and veggies first) is for blood sugar stabilization, satiety, recovery from training, hormone production, health, muscle growth and maintenance. So that's all you really need to know about WHY it is important. Protein is PRIORITY.

We get the majority of our protein needs from healthy animal sources. Remember, "If it had a mom, it's a protein." This means wild caught fish (salmon, cod, etc.), grass-fed beef (steak, ground beef), healthy chicken sources (breast, thigh, ground, sausage), turkey (breast, thigh, ground, sausage), pork, eggs, lamb, shellfish, and other animal sources.

I say HEALTHY animal sources because some factory farmed sources are extremely unhealthy. Factory farmed fish like tilapia are fed grains instead of their natural food source, have chemicals and antibiotics put in the water they live in, which means YOU are eating chemicals and antibiotics if you eat them. Yuck. So always get "wild caught" fish. Check the frozen and fresh sections of your grocery store to ensure that what you buy is what you should eat.

The same applies to beef. Regular factory farmed beef is full of hormones, antibiotics and they too are fed an unnatural food source, usually corn, which is not their natural food source so the meat is low quality and unhealthy. ALWAYS get "organic grass-fed" beef, because it's healthier, has no antibiotics, no hormones, tastes better, and has more nutrients. Make sure you invest in quality protein like you do quality clothes, shoes, home, and cars.

We have covered the importance of protein, so let's move to the other very important macro, FAT.

Fats

Thanks to the biggest mistake in nutritional history back in 1977, fat has gotten a bad rap in relation to heart disease and weight gain. Like I mentioned earlier in this book, fats are the macro that was once thought caused heart disease and obesity, so the government launched the low-fat era. Food companies started taking the fats out of foods, but when you do that, it tastes like cardboard, so they started pumping in sugar and flour. This mistake is what has led to severe sugar addiction, obesity epidemic, and our chronic disease epidemic.

Look around you. Everyone is overweight, obese, and eats trash all day. Next time you go to the grocery store, look inside the grocery carts of the typical American and obese person. You will see cake, cookies, soda, processed foods, yogurts, sweetened drinks, bread, pasta, and a ton of other highly addictive, fat promoting foods. This mistake is why Americans are now so fat and sick.

This generation of kids – YOUR kids – are actually expected to die BEFORE their parents. This is because the parents started their children's lives off with the same awful eating habits they have today. This is why today's kids are getting fatter and developing disease at much younger ages. And all of this is because of the low-fat era.

But it turns out, fats weren't ever the enemy at all. We took the fat out of foods and we got FATTER and SICKER. Fats weren't the problem; it was primarily processed food, sugar, flour, that were causing obesity and heart disease. These low-fat guidelines have cost millions of people their lives. We have ALL lost loved ones because of these diseases. We have even lost some due to this low-fat era. From diabetes, heart disease, cancer, Alzheimer's (dubbed Diabetes Type 3), stroke, these are ALL diet-related, lifestyle caused diseases. Foods that spike blood sugar like sugar, flour, and processed foods are the primary cause.

Fats are not the enemy. Good fats are good friends. There are some bad ones, like trans-fats, processed vegetable oils, but these are generally found in processed foods and restaurant foods. Eliminate processed foods and poor choices at restaurants and you fully avoid the bad fats. Fats aren't what makes you fat, they actually help you get FIT! We NEED them.

What foods are considered fats?

Good fat sources are unrefined animal fats, select plant fats, and oils. Saturated fats are also a necessary component of our biology. These fats include almonds, bacon, avocados, egg yolks, grass-fed butter (yep, its approved), coconut oil, olive oil, meats, and fish have excellent sources of good fats. So what exactly are fats and why do we need them?

Science: Fats are known as triglycerides and fatty acids. They are one of the three macronutrients that are vital to the bodily processes such as digestion, transport, conversion, and energy. There are nine calories for every gram, which is the MOST calorie-dense out of all three macros, as proteins and carbs are four calories per gram.

Fats are essential for health, wellbeing and is NECESSARY for many reasons.

"Your body requires a good amount of fats in your diet to stay lean."
-Charles Poliquin

- Eating a greater proportion of your calories from fat will help you achieve a shredded physique.

- Fat makes up the outside layer of ALL of the cells in your body. Did you hear that? It makes up the outside layer of ALL cells. Muscles are CELLS.

- By decreasing carb intake and replacing it with fat intake, you can improve your utilization of insulin, reduce inflammation, and support your metabolism.

- Omega 3's help turn on genes that are involved with burning fat, while turning off the genes that store fat. They also support thyroid hormone function which is involved your body fat regulation. Just think of fish oil, as it is high in Omega 3's.

- Fat is filling! When eaten with protein, fat can lead to more satiety and satisfaction. It keeps you fuller longer.

- Fat helps with muscle growth because it supports hormonal balance.

- A diet higher in fat can also elevate growth hormone.

- Fat is used to manufacture hormones. Hormones NEED fats to be adequately developed.

- Fat increases libido.

- Fat is essential for the absorption of certain vitamins.

- Your brain is composed of around 60% fats.

- Dietary fat is an excellent energy source.

Fat is a pretty important macro, huh? Fuvk yes! This is one of the missing links in a lot of the current physique athletes, bodybuilders, competitors. They tend to do the old-school, higher carb, lower fat type of diet. This is also part of the reason why most of them binge or rebound, post show or photoshoot. It's also one of the reasons why they get super crazy and grumpy while dieting. If they actually had adequate fats throughout the year, they would LOOK awesome and FEEL awesome all year.

The BEST Fat: Essential Fatty Acids (EFSs) Omega 3's

Essential fatty acids cannot be manufactured by the body, so they need to be obtained from the diet. These essentials are Omega 3 and 6, but we get plenty of Omega 6 through our diet and so we don't need to increase our intake of those, but we need to pay special attention to increasing our intake of Omega 3. Most people are severely deficient in Omega 3 and aren't even aware. So our focus is to increase our Omega 3 intake for our bodies to function optimally so we can LOOK amazing.

Why is Omega 3 so important?

Omega 3 plays a vital role in many cellular functions, they affect EVERY part of your biochemistry. They control gene function, regulate your immune system, impact the speed and efficacy of your metabolism and they are a vital component of the cell membrane that covers every one of the 100 trillion cells in your body.

Think they're important? Fuvk YESSS!!!

This means when you don't get enough Omega 3, it can contribute to excess inflammation in the body, raising risks to certain health issues. Messages can't be properly communicated from one cell to another. It leads to poor brain function, anxiety, depression, skin disorders, digestive disorders, and your body not functioning at its full potential.

Omega 3 is the MOST important FAT. But being that most people don't eat nearly enough fish to get adequate Omega 3, it is best to supplement them with fish oil in a capsule or liquid form. Even if you eat quite a bit of fish, you're probably still deficient.

I recommend 10 to 20 grams of fish oil per day minimum. Yes, that means 10 to 20 pills, or a couple tablespoons of oil per day. You'll be surprised how much better you look and feel when you have adequate Omega 3 in your diet, so Omega 3 up!!!

We covered two of the three macros, and now it's time to talk about everyone's favorite macro: CARBS.

Carbs: The world's favorite macro

Carbs are often pointed as the enemy of burning fat and getting shredded, but you actually DO need carbs in your diet – just not as much as you would like. Most people prioritize their carb intake and overeat them on a daily basis, which is why everyone is so fat.

When you eat carbs, they are broken down in your system into blood sugar. Depending on how many grams you ate and the type of carbs will determine how fast your blood sugar rises. Your pancreas secretes insulin to remove excess blood sugar from your blood because high blood sugar is toxic. Its job is to deposit it into your muscles, and liver, but if your muscle and liver stores are FULL it gets stored as FAT. Insulin is a storage hormone, and anything in excess carbs and calories, get stored as fat. One of the keys to getting shredded is keeping your insulin levels in check.

Having insulin in your blood stream blunts fat burning. So keeping insulin levels in check, by controlling your carb intake is key to getting shredded. Good times to eat carbs are right before or after your workouts. After your workouts when some of your glycogen stores are depleted, the insulin response to carbs will deposit the carbs and other nutrients into your muscles. Carbs eaten before training will be utilized to train.

Carbs come in many different forms, and they all have a different effect on your blood sugar. Most people when they hear the word "carbs" think of the processed foods like bread, pasta, rice, chips, sweets, and soda. These types of carbs have been refined, processed, the fiber has been removed, have added sugar or flour, and it is digested INSTANTLY. They cause a higher blood sugar spike and a subsequent blood sugar crash after insulin has done its job.

Most people who eat these types of foods go through these cycles of blood sugar spikes and crashes, constantly which another aspect that makes them crave more carbs and leads to body fat gain. Yes this even applies to whole-wheat bread; it's trash as well, thanks to the scientific engineering of crops today.

Why carbs have a bad rap

The reason why carbs have been pointed as the enemy is because most people eat the WRONG ones DAILY and these are the ones responsible for everyone being fat and sick. The ones I'm speaking of are the processed, refined, manmade ones that contain sugar and flour. These are the TRUE enemy.

Do you remember why they are the enemy? Let's review real quick:

1.   **Addiction.** These types of foods are eight times more addictive than cocaine. Because they are so ADDICTIVE most people have one bite and then binge. These foods trigger a release of dopamine in the brain that make you FEEL good (you confuse it with tasting good), which leads to you eating MORE than you should at that meal. It also will trigger cravings the rest of that day, the day after that and the day after that. So this leads to you overeating and getting fatter.

2.   **Fat Storing.** These foods also spike your blood sugar rapidly, leading to a burst of insulin (fat storing hormone). Insulin has a few things it does, from causing a blood sugar CRASH, storing any excess blood glucose (what carbs convert to once eaten), inhibits fat breakup and the production of fat-burning hormones. The blood sugar crash will lead to you wanting a nap, craving MORE carbs/sugar to feel better and bring blood sugar back up. This leads to even more overeating, more blood sugar spikes, insulin bursts, fat storing, crashing, and craving it once again. It's a vicious cycle that people mindlessly put themselves through daily.

3.   **Systemic Inflammation.** Foods containing flour, sugar, processed oils, or that are highly processed or refined damage your gut health, cause leaky gut, and lead to systemic inflammation. This is the number one reason people get diagnosed with autoimmune diseases, depression, skin issues like eczema, psoriasis, and every other disease you can imagine is linked to leaky gut and inflammation.

But the reason why this is also bad is because it causes muscle and joint pain. This means that when you train, something is going to hurt and you're going to be limited and not be able to perform your best. Which means sucky workout for you and less results, so now you're days behind where you should be in a few weeks – all from five minutes of glory of some processed crap. NOT WORTH IT!

This is why we don't do cheat meals. This is why we don't do IIFYM, or "flexible dieting." A lot of coaches today still promote and allow their clients "cheat meals" weekly, and most of these coaches have clients that are always in pain, just look average, or keep high body fat year-round. On top of that, most coaches have limited, if any, nutritional education whatsoever. They are clueless about blood sugar, insulin, food addiction, inflammation, or any of that. Truly, they just don't know about it, which is why they still allow cheat meals.

But these cheat meals are killing their clients' hard work, their self-esteem, leading to frustration, and killing client retention. Occasionally, you find the exception to this, once in a while you'll find a ripped client that does get away with weekly cheat meals, but these are RARE super-disciplined people. I guarantee they are inflamed and working around injuries constantly. But for 99.999% of people in America, it's these cheat meals that are WHY they stay average, fat, and always in pain.

We don't do average. Fuvk average. We do OutFuvkingStanding and piss on average! Which is why we don't do cheat meals.

Why I oppose IIFYM (flexible dieting)

It is because of the reasons I stated above that are why I'm opposed to IIFYM style dieting, or "flexible dieting." It is a form of dieting that uses processed foods to achieve some of the macros. For example, eating Pop Tarts instead of a banana for your carbs or eating cereal instead of a bowl of strawberries for your carbs. This is known as IIFYM (if it fits your macros) a/k/a flexible dieting.

Although this sounds great to your inner food ADDICT, it does not work for 99.99% of the population. It takes EXTREME self-discipline to utilize this type of lifestyle, which most people DO NOT have. Due to the extreme addiction of the processed foods, most people cannot stop at one Pop Tart or 155 grams of ice cream, so it leads to addictive behaviors. This leads to a binge, which leads to overeating, which leads to excess body fat. Then it leads to inflammation and you having to work around an injury. It's not worth it.

In today's social media world, I'm sure you've seen the people bragging about their brownies and candy they use for their carbs. But what you don't see are the aches and pains that they have or the injuries they have accumulated or are working around. You don't see the drugs they use, which give them the extra edge, to get 10 times more results with a fraction of the work. You don't see that some of them are truly on point and eat flawless the majority of the time, then have their treat once in a while.

You don't see them struggle with cravings afterward, either. You don't see that most of these people are usually chubbier most of the year, except when it's time for a physique show or photoshoot. You don't see what may be going on inside their bodies that may show up later in the future as cancer or other long-term effects. Why risk it? Just feed your body NATURAL foods and you avoid all the possible downsides.

Hell, you may be one of these models/coaches reading this book right now and haven't connected the dots to your cravings, binging, fat gaining, and injuries until now. Well, now you know. You're welcome, coaches. Now help me and help the world transform by promoting EATING REAL FOOD!

So enough about processed carbs. What kinds of foods are considered carbs that are healthy whole food sources?

Did you know that VEGGIES are carbs? Yep, it's true.

Did you know that fruit are carbs? Yep, that's true too.

Did you know that oats, quinoa, beans, and rice are also carbs? Yep, that's true too!

Carbs that get you shredded

The only approved carbs you are allowed to eat are those that come from NATURE: the ones that came from a plant – mainly veggies, veggies, veggies and some fruit. These are the ones that provide fiber, micronutrients (vitamins, minerals), health, and energy. These also aren't addictive like processed carbs, so you won't have intense cravings after consuming them. You can literally EAT AS MANY veggies as you want! Hungry? Eat more veggies! (The low-carb ones.)

How many people have you ever met that got fat from eating kale, broccoli, cauliflower, spinach, and asparagus? NONE! These are filling and aren't addictive. You would be so full from eating lots of these that you would end up eating LESS calories the rest of the day. I DARE you to eat as much broccoli as you can until you're full. I bet you don't eat the rest of the day, and maybe even half the next day.

Know that you may not like the taste of some veggies at first and there is no magic solution you have to retrain your taste buds to enjoy them. When you clean up your diet, it can take up to three weeks for your palate to change. Once it does, you will start to taste the flavor of them more and enjoy them more.

Although raw veggies are always best, I personally do most of my veggies steamed, or sautéed, this brings out their flavor more, so feel free to experiment.

Quick list of carb sources.

Fruit: Bananas, apples, oranges, pears, berries, etc.
Veggies: Broccoli, asparagus, lettuce, kale, spinach, cauliflower, etc.
Grains: Oats, beans, rice, quinoa etc.

You will be eating carbs every meal, every day, primarily in veggie form. But you will have the other carb sources in your nutrition as well.

Benefits of healthy carbs

-   They increase your fiber intake to aid in excellent digestion.
-   Veggies help keep blood sugar stable, which is key to fat loss.
-   They keep you feeling fuller longer, which leads to less overall hunger and calorie consumption.
-   They provide micronutrients (vitamins, minerals) to your body, which are the raw materials it needs to function optimally.
-   They provide good, clean energy.
-   They provide antioxidants.

- They don't have addictive components and don't trigger cravings.

So I'm sure you get the picture: cut the crap carbs (sugar, flour, processed foods) and eat the good ones that came straight from a PLANT (veggies, fruit, quinoa, etc.).

Now that we have discussed macros, let's move on to understanding HOW your body works and HOW we are going to get it to burn fat so you get shredded!

Eating healthy isn't good enough

Kicking the sugar habit and committing to eating only REAL whole foods is only the part of the process. This alone will make dramatic changes in your body, metabolism and health. But to get SHREDDED, you have to take it another couple steps further.

How do you know how much 6 oz. of chicken is, or 1 Tbsp. of olive oil, or 100 g of a banana is? How do you know if that was ½ or ¾ cup? How do you know what 14 g of peanut butter is?

Do you eyeball it? Guesstimate? Fuvk no!

You WEIGH your portions. Yes, on a food scale. And yes, this is necessary. Cleaning up your diet is the first step, but controlling your portions is the next one. To create accuracy in your intake, you have to weigh your portions. This is a MUST! Otherwise, you are wasting your time working out because you are not going to get the body you want. You're not going to get shredded at the rate you want, or even EVER, and you will not develop muscle the way you're supposed to if your portions and macros aren't right.

By weighing your portions, you will get the appropriate macros and calories, which creates the right response(deficit) and recovery we seek.

Nutrition is 80% of fat loss

Some professionals will even say it's more like 90%. But regardless of whatever it is, it's the MOST vital element to you getting shredded and adding muscle. So if nutrition is the most vital element, what does that mean you need to MASTER? Your nutrition! Yes or yes?

To get to the body you want, your nutrition has to be ON Fuvking POINT seven days a week! How many days a week? 7 days a week!

Okay, so you know nutrition is 80% of your results. You know you have to master it and you know that you have to weigh portions. But what's the next step?

How do you know what your macros are for the day?

How do you know how many calories you've eaten?

How do you know the macros for the 6 oz. of chicken, or how many carbs are in 100 g of banana?

How do you know when you are done eating for the day?

How do you find out?

You track it!

The only way you are going to know where you stand, how many calories you have eaten, or the macros in your foods, or know when you are DONE eating for the day, is by tracking EVERY bite you consume.

Everything has calories, and everything adds up and everything counts. You MUST weigh the correct portions, and you MUST track every bite to get shredded.

Technology makes it easy

Back in the day we used to do this with pen and paper, but thanks to the advances in technology, there are apps that do all the work for you. All you have to do is select the proper food, the proper serving size, and it does all the math for you. Simple! I personally used to do this with pen and paper, and it was effective, but it was also a little time consuming. Lucky for you now, we have apps and websites at our disposal.

Two times more success

Some studies have shown that those who track are two times more successful than people who don't. TWO times! Do you want double the results or would you like to get shredded two times faster than the average guy? Hell yes! Sign me up! The app we use is called MyFitnessPal. Look it up on your smartphone and download it NOW. This is the app I recommend all my clients and I personally use it as well. It's even so awesome that Under Armor apparel bought MyFitnessPal for $475,000,000 not too long ago. WOW!

Why do we track? Why does it deliver such incredible results? Good question. It does a few things, but the primary reasons, are self-awareness and personal accountability.

Awareness

By weighing and tracking your portions, you are going to be made more aware of exactly how many grams of protein, carbs, fats, and calories you have eaten. You are also going to know how many calories, or macros you have remaining, and you are going to know when you are done for the day. When you start tracking your intake, you will quickly find how fast these calories add up, you will find out that what you were eating was A LOT more calorie-dense, or high in carbs than you thought. You will start to be more aware of what you eat, be more aware of the choices you make, be more conscious of food. The more aware and conscious you are of your intake, the better your nutrition is.

Accountability

Another aspect to the awareness is it's a way to hold yourself accountable. "Before you smack it, you better track it." By knowing that every bite you eat is going to be logged and SHOW in writing, you are more likely to be accountable to your actions. To eat something, you HAVE to track it.

By knowing you have to track it, you will more than likely choose to NOT eat that extra bite, or poor food choice because you won't want to fail or see it in writing. It's amazing how that works, huh? This is self-accountability. I can't be there to slap the food out of your mouth, so you have to have the integrity and discipline to do it yourself. Awareness and accountability are key elements to you getting shredded.

Your nutrition has to be your number one focus every day. The only way all of your hard work, sweat, time, effort, and tears are going pay off in the mirror is by you MASTERING your nutrition. By weighing and tracking your intake and hitting your daily macro/calorie requirements, you are guaranteed to get shredded. These two tools are your training partners, your best friends that are going to deliver abs to your doorstep. Utilize them!

Be obsessed

"If you don't have the mental capacity to be obsessed about what you are trying to get, then muthafuvker you aren't ever going to get it."
–CT Fletcher

Just like achieving your goals in business and finances, you have to OBSESS yourself over your nutrition and training. If people aren't telling you, "You're crazy. You're obsessed. You're a maniac," then that means you are putting in average effort. If average people aren't commenting, talking crap, then you're not putting in the level of effort that is required to succeed. You have to put in obsessive efforts to succeed in getting shredded.

When you are at that level, when you rise above mediocrity, the average peasants will bark and complain. This is a good sign you are headed in the right direction. So be obsessed about what goes in your mouth. Always know exactly what you are getting from your food. Be obsessed about training DAILY. You have to obsess over your food intake, obsess over your training each and every day. They are a priority, everything else comes second. When you take care of YOU first, everything else will fall into place. Shredded is a lifestyle, and living shredded requires absolute obsession!

So GET OBSESSED! Seek comments from the peasants. It's a good sign.

Don't be a 'lil bitch

This journey of getting shredded is not easy. I just told you, you are going to have to be obsessed about your food intake, obsessed about your training. So you are going to have to man the fuvk up and don't be a little bitch. You will have peasants talk crap and you will have people trying to talk you down, but this is life. You will also be surrounded by addictive junk foods every day, at every social event, and at every dinner. So what? You are going to have to man up, stand your ground and do what's right and what's best for you.

"Don't be a lil bitch" means don't give in. Don't let the peasants persuade you. Don't be undisciplined. Don't be weak. You are a MAN, so ACT like one. Men are dominant. Men are masculine. Men are in control. Be a fuvking MAN!

Now that you are obsessed, now that you are manning the fuvk up, it's time for your tools!

Get your shredder tools!

Shredder Tool #1: A food scale. Buy a digital food scale that weighs in ounces and grams. You can find them online, at Walmart, Target, or even at some grocery stores. There is no magic brand; just make sure it is digital and weighs in grams and ounces. These are usually around $20, give or take a few dollars, so go get one NOW!

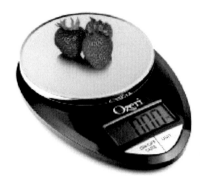

Shredder Tool #2. MyFitnessPal app.

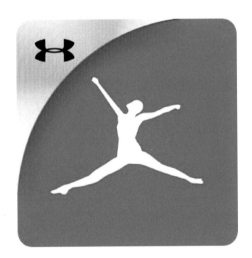

If you haven't already, download the MyFitnessPal app and set up your profile. Keep in mind, I am going to give you your recommended calorie/macros in a moment. So DO NOT FOLLOW the calories or macros the app recommends.

Also, do NOT track your workouts on this app, because it will change your calories and macros. Just download and set it up. I will give you recommendations shortly.

You can also login online from your computer at www.myfitnesspal.com. Don't worry, I have made it simple. Just know that in order to be accurate with your intake and create the proper environment for change, you MUST use those two tools.

Let's review:

1. What is the biggest nutritional mistake in history?
2. What is responsible for our obesity and chronic disease
3. epidemic?
4. Why is it addictive?
5. How addictive is it?
6. How do you kick the habit?
7. What day is the peak day of detox?
8. What do most people say by Day 7?
9. What is the only kind of food you should eat?
10. What is real food?
11. What does PVF mean?
12. What is the belief I recommended you adopt?
13. Besides addiction, cravings, body fat, what does processed food cause?
14. What are the only foods allowed in your kitchen?
15. What are macros?
16. Why is protein so important?
17. Why are fats so important?
18. What carbs can you eat TONS of?
19. Why aren't calories created equal
20. What are three proteins, three fats, and three carbs?

21. What's the most important fat?
22. Why don't we do cheat meals?
23. What are the two Shredder Tools?
24. "You need to be ____" to succeed.
25. "Don't be a lil _____"

[7]

How to Get Shredded

Understanding your body

Would you like to know how your body works?
Would you like to learn HOW to get the body to burn fat?
Then pay attention.

Your BMR

Do you know what your BMR stands for? In order to get shredded, there are a few things you must understand about your body and metabolism. BMR stands for your Basal Metabolic Rate, which is the amount of calories your body uses/burns daily just to function and survive. Your body burns calories 24/7; it's like a car running at idle while you sit and sleep. It's like a car hitting the throttle when you're training. It requires energy and fuel ALL day to function.

It requires energy for your brain to function, your digestion, body heat, heartbeat, and all the other cellular and bodily functions you never even think about. All of these functions require calories, like a car engine that never turns off. Your body is ALWAYS melting calories. Always.

Your BMR is very important and is where the majority of your calories burned each day come from. The more muscle you have, the taller you are, the HIGHER your BMR. The higher your BMR is, the faster you burn fat. This is one of the reasons why taller, more muscular men get shredded faster. This is one of the reasons why men burn fat faster than women. Higher BMRs lead to higher overall calories burned.

Let's take Average Joe for instance. Joe is a 5'9" 195 lb. man. He is an average looking guy, has a typical desk job, works out a few times a week, but doesn't really look like it. This is about the average height, weight, and lifestyle of most men in America. Joe may have a BMR of around 2,000 calories, which is the amount of calories his body burns daily just to function and keep him alive.

So if he was a lazy ass and laid in bed all day, he would burn a minimum of 2,000 calories. This is where the greatest amount of your energy expenditure and calorie burn comes from, so we want to protect it, and develop it. We protect it and develop it by training hard, training effectively, and making sure we are eating CORRECTLY. You want to always FEED your muscles so you can maintain them, and improve your BMR by developing more muscle.

Total Daily Energy Expenditure (TDEE)

Now you know where the majority of your calorie burn comes from, now what is the TDEE? This is the total amount of calories your body burns in a 24-hour period. This is your BMR plus sleeping, working, working out, walking around, playing, sexual activities, sports, and even digesting food! This means we ALWAYS burn more than our BMR, unless you're bedridden (which you may be sometimes after one of our Leg Days). But even then you'll still burn more calories than your BMR from the "afterburn" and recovery effect from Leg Day.

TDEE is the most important factor when determining your caloric intake to gain muscle or get shredded. Which we will cover in a bit. But know that your TDEE is basically your total caloric burn for the day. This level of calories is the starting point on where we decide what your calories should be.

For example, Joe's BMR is around 2,000 calories. But when you add in his daily activities plus workout, his total energy expenditure for the day (his total calories burned) will be around 3,000 or more calories.

In my 13 years of training, the one thing that I have noticed is that based off of your height, weight, age, and activity, men are generally within just a few 100 calories of each other in terms of intake needs to maintain muscle and burn fat. For years, I used to use certain websites and formulas to establish calorie intake and macros. However, after writing up hundreds of plans, I realized that each person is only within a few hundred calories of each other based on their height, weight, and activity.

So instead of giving you some crazy, confusing formula or math equation, I created an awesome simplified system of how to determine recommended intakes for EVERYONE. You will read this later on. What I have found is that the average guys needs to burn fat and get shredded ranges between 2,100 and 2,500 calories per day, depending on his physical stats and activity.

Average Joe at 5'9" and 196 pounds may need about 2,200 calories to get shredded.

John at 6'3" and 225 pounds may need 2,500 or more.

This is only a few hundred calories difference, which is why I'm going to be giving you example meal plans and calorie recommendations later on to simplify this for you. Your goal each day is to get your TDEE (total calorie burn) as high as possible, to create more of a deficit. Now let's talk about HOW to get shredded by creating a "deficit."

What getting shredded is

What is getting shredded? Do you really know what being shredded really is? The reason I ask this is because most people have no clue what it takes or what being shredded really is. I ask this question all the time to new clients and you should hear some of the ridiculous answers I get.

Just so you can get it straight and understood, I'm going to tell you. Getting toned, defined, losing weight, getting ripped, getting shredded, what you're seeking is ALL the same thing: FAT LOSS. I mention this because magazines and TV tends to confuse people by the words they use to target specific markets. Getting shredded is purely losing fat and getting to very low body fat levels. That's it. Anyone wanting to get "toned, ripped, defined, lose weight, and get shredded" are all ultimately seeking the same exact thing: burning fat!

You already have abs, you already have the lines in the arms, legs, chest and back musculature, and you already have the striations in the muscles. Even if you don't work out, you already have it; this is how the muscles are formed, how the body is shaped, and everyone has it. You just can't see it because you have a thick layer of fat covering it. Get the fat off and get to low body fat levels, then you will reveal the muscles and start looking "defined". This is how you get the look that is known as SHREDDED.

That's it. This is not a special kind of diet, type of training, or a special pill. It is simply getting your macros on point, training hard, burning fat, and TIME. That's all it takes to get your body fat so low you appear shredded. This is common sense, but I feel I should reiterate it. It takes anywhere from 8-20+ weeks for the average person to get shredded, depending on where they started.

So what causes the body to burn fat?

Burning fat comes from DIET + intense WEIGHT training, leading to a deficit – NOT tons of cardio. As matter of fact, if your diet is dialed in and your weight training is intense, you don't have to do ANY CARDIO to get shredded. PERIOD. You're not going to be doing one to two hours of cardio per day like the old-school, outdated coaches teach. That is muscle wasting, time wasting, and testosterone reducing.

Remember, what is responsible for 80% of your fat loss?

The most important thing you need to be focusing on to get shredded is your DIET. Your DIET is where 80% of your results come from. Eighty percent! That means you can be doing the most badass workouts for hours per week(which we have in this book), but if your diet isn't on point, neither will be your results. That is why I am spending so much time trying to educate you about food. Vice versa, the MORE dialed-in your nutrition, the LESS work you have to do. You're still going to have to work your ass off, but a lot less when your diet is on point.

So if nutrition is 80% of your fat loss results, what should your focus be on? What should you master? Your focus should be to get your "Diet ON POINT. DIET dialed in. Every damn day, seven days a week." – Daymond Sewall

How to get shredded

"The hour spent training in the gym is important, but it's how you spend the other 23 that determine your results." - Unknown

Now that you understand your BMR and TDEE, I can explain how to get the body to burn fat so you can get shredded as fuvk and look like a god! Do you know what makes the body burn fat? Do you know WHY the body gains fat?

There are 7 billion people on the planet, and all of our bodies work exactly the same. Some to greater degrees than others, but for the most part they work exactly the same in theory. The body stores fat for one purpose and the body burns fat for one purpose. You have heard this a thousand times before, but I'm going to break it down dummy-style so it makes sense.

So what makes the body burn fat?

The only way your body will burn fat is if it is FORCED to burn fat, and the only way the human body will dig into its fat stores if if you create a "calorie deficit". This means eating slightly less than you burn or burning more than you consume. Whichever way you want to look at it, it's the same. When you do this, this is known as creating a "caloric deficit." I personally have dubbed the term "deficiting," used like "I am deficiting!" or, "You better be deficiting!"

Creating a calorie deficit is the ONLY way the human body will dig into its fat stores. Fat is basically an extra fuel tank for your bodies energy requirements. It does not want to burn it and it does not want to let it go. You have to create the proper environment (deficit) to force it to dig into its stored energy. We create the deficit by eating a specific amount of macros, when you hit your prescribed macros you will achieve the desired caloric limit, that creates calorie deficit to burn fat. Simple, huh? It is, it just takes discipline.

How the body gains fat

So if creating a calorie deficit is how you burn fat, how did you gain fat? By the exact opposite process, you ate MORE than your body burned, so it stored the excess as fat. Just like if you try and top of your car's gas tank, the fuel spills out all over the ground, that's how your body fat is. That extra spillover gets stored for later into your amazingly disgusting fat cells. Got fat? You've overeaten on many, many, many occasions.

One bad day can set you back a week. This is why learning to master your weekends is key to getting consistent results week by week. Get your macros on point every day of the week, not just five.

Example of a calorie deficit

Average Joe is 5'9" and 195 pounds. On a day he trains hard, his body is going to burn 3,000+ calories that day. This includes his BMR (Basal Metabolic Rate), which is the amount of calories required to sustain life, breathing heart rate, body temp, etc. His BMR is approximately 2,000 calories. Add in his workout and recovery from previous workouts, and he's burning about 3,000 calories a day.

The ONLY way his body will burn fat is if he is in a DEFICIT, eating LESS than he burns. So if Joe only eats 2,200 calories (deficit) but burns 3,000, his body is then FORCED to dig into fat stores to make up the 800 calorie deficit. 3,000 − 2,200 =

800 fat calories burned. This is how you manipulate your body to burn fat. This is also the ONLY way the human body will burn fat.

FYI: 3,500 calories = 1 pound of fat. Do this for six days straight and that's over 1.3 pounds of fat burned, by the linear math equation. This is how you burn fat. This done consistently is how you get shredded. This is why we have to weigh and track EVERYTHING. It's the only way you know whether or not you are in a deficit, or you have overeaten. Really, it's to prevent you from overeating and keep you in check.

Never go over your limit

What do you do when you hit your calorie goal? By weighing portions and tracking your intake on MyFitnessPal, you are going to know exactly where your calories and macros are. When your calories have been met, you're DONE. I don't care if it's 1:00 p.m. in the afternoon and you go to bed at 10:00 p.m. Drink water and take your ass to bed. Never go over your calorie goal limits – as a matter of fact, I'd like for you to be just a hair under them. You HAVE to stay under your calorie limits and KEEP your deficit so you melt fat, period.

When you're done, you're DONE. Drink water. Suck it up and take your ass to bed. Keep your deficit! You will wake up leaner, with more self-confidence from your small accomplishment of being disciplined.

You may have days where you are hungrier

What do you do on days you're hungrier? When your body is in a deficit, burning fat, it sometimes triggers hunger. Remember, it doesn't want to burn fat and it wants to keep it, so it may send some hunger signals. Or you may have days where you hit your calorie limit very early in the day because you ate very calorie-dense foods early on.

So what do you do? You suck it up, Princess! Your ass starves until the next day. Keep your deficit! Guzzle water. You will wake up with more results.

Three things that cause hunger

Want to know three things that cause hunger that you may not know?

Dehydration. When you are dehydrated your body can sometimes trigger hunger. So if you ever feel hunger, ask yourself, "How much water have I consumed? When was the last time I peed?"

Nine times out of 10, you will find you are dehydrated. A quick hydration test is to just think about when the last time you peed. If you haven't done it in the last 20 minutes, you're dehydrated, in my opinion. Your pee should be frequent and clear/almost clear. If it is not, you're dehydrated. So guzzle up 20-40 ounces of water immediately!

Sodium depletion. If you haven't been getting an adequate amount of salt (Himalayan salt or sea salt) in your diet, you're going to feel like shit with all of the intense training. Make sure you add salt to food, and add ½ tsp. of salt or more, before training and after training. If you ever feel an energy dip during training, that's also a sign of dehydration or need for salt. That's just a little secret of mine. I keep salt in my gym bag.

Fat Burning. If your water is good, sodium is good, macros are good, and you're still hungry, then it's just your body burning fat. Suck it up! Drink more water and fill your belly up.

Know your limits

Each day you're going to have limits on your calorie intake, so DO NOT go above them. Your deficit days have limits and your REFEED(high calorie) days have limits. This is to keep you burning fat on deficit days, and to keep you from storing fat on refeed days. We will discuss refeed days in a bit.

The human body is a complex system

The human body is different than inside a lab or in black and white. It is said that one pound of fat burned in a lab would give you an estimated 3,500 calories of energy. But when it comes to the body there are many hormones, metabolic processes, and other factors that come into play. So when it comes to the body burning fat, I have found that it actually comes much faster than what the simple linear math of these numbers say, but you get the idea.

The ONLY thing you need to know is to keep your diet on point and you will burn fat. Know that the ONLY way your body will burn fat is if you create a deficit, even if you're eating 100% healthy. This means Average Joe could be eating 100% whole, real food, but if he eats 3,000 calories or more, he's not going to lose crap.

Now do you see why weighing your portions and obsessively tracking your intake is crucial to your success?

Nutrition is 80% of your results, the only way all your sweat, blood, tears and time invested will pay off from the gym, is if your diet is ON POINT. Just like how sales is the most important element of your business, NUTRITION is the most important element of the business of getting shredded.

It's NOT your genetics

"No deficit, no loss. Period."
-Daymond Sewall

One thing I have found that is very common in most people is that they often play the victim in life and especially with their bodies. Now being that you're an executive/entrepreneur in business or in your life, this is probably not you, but just in case this topic needs to be discussed. You see, most people say they are working out and eating better, but their body isn't losing weight or burning fat like they expect it to, they are always quick to point blame at their BODY for not responding.

Do you know that person? The one that ACTS like they are doing it all right, but they are still fat? They say things like, "I don't know what's going on. I'm eating healthy, working out, but I just can't lose any weight. I'm doing everything right but the scale isn't moving. Why can't I lose any weight?"

Yea, you know that person, its hopefully NOT you, but before it continues or becomes you, I'm going to bitch slap you with some TRUTH.

What did we just discuss about WHY the body burns fat? If you're not burning fat or losing as fast as you like, know that it's not your thyroid, it's not your hormones, it's not your age, it's not your genetics, it's not a slow metabolism, it's not the air, wind, sun, or pollution. It's NOT starvation mode!

It's not any one of these or anything else you want to point blame, IT'S YOU. If you aren't losing, what are you not doing? You're NOT creating a deficit! You're not creating a deficit, so your body has no reason to burn fat. It's not your body and it's not your genetics. You are simply OVERCONSUMING.

Getting shredded is more than just "eating right" or "eating healthy." I just gave you an example in the last section but in case you missed it...

You can eat healthy and still consume 4,000 calories per day. Let's say you trained legs and burned a total of 3,000 calories today, but you ate 4,000 calories of healthy food. What do you think is going to happen? Your extra 1,000 calories consumed just went straight to body fat – straight to your muffin top.

If you aren't losing fat, then that's proof you are not weighing portions and tracking your food consistently. That's your first problem. We already discussed this in previous sections. But If you're not weighing your portions and tracking your intake, how the fuvk do you think you're going to know how many calories you ate? How are you going to know when you have hit your limit and you're done? How do you expect to get results when you're not doing the fuvking work?! Nutrition is 80%!

Your lack of results are telling you that you're NOT in a deficit. Your lack of fat loss is saying YOU'RE EATING TOO MUCH. *No deficit, No loss. Period.* If you create a deficit you will lose 100% of the time. Yes, I said 100% of the time!

No deficit, no...?

No loss! Yes, healthy food can make you fat. Yes, healthy food can also prevent you from losing fat if you eat too much. Now if you are actually weighing and tracking, yet still aren't losing, then what may be happening is you are miscalculating or tracking the WRONG food selection on the app. Either way, if you're not losing fat consistently, that means you're not creating a deficit to burn fat. So figure out what it is you're doing wrong and FIX it.

No deficit, no loss. Period.

It's NOT starvation mode

This is a COMMON misconception, which is why I'm covering this topic. People tend to try and blame their lack of fat loss on starvation mode. This mode is supposedly their body's response to them not eating frequently enough or enough calories. The theory is that they are skipping meals and not eating frequently enough so their metabolism instantly shuts down and hoards their fat. They aren't feeding the body often enough, so the body just stops burning calories. Heard of that before? Sounds familiar? Well its HORSE SHIT!

Your body isn't going to shut down your metabolism and just stop burning because you didn't feed it often enough or ate too few calories. We already discussed this. Your body is ALWAYS running and always burning calories just to maintain survival, just like that car running at idle. It IS NOT your body being a little bitch and slowing your metabolism because you underfed it or went to long without eating. This theory is BS! You are just not creating a deficit. You are overeating and/or not training hard enough.

No deficit, no loss. Period. Your body is going to continue burning at near the same rate whether you feed it or not. It is not going to just quickly shut down. We would have become extinct long ago if that was the case.

But what will happen if it feels starved, if you under eat, or stay in a deficit for extremely long periods is that it will change its energy source. If you go long periods where the body is severely underfed or too long in deficit, it may feel threatened, and for survival purposes, it slows down the utilization of fat for energy and instead starts to utilize MUSCLE. But the burning continues and will be at an equivalent rate; it's just coming from a different energy source. Your metabolism doesn't just shut down because you didn't feed it. It will still run but just off of a different fuel.

What's really happening

I have found that those who always claim "starvation mode" as their excuse tend to be the ones who go long periods of time without eating. They are the ones who skip breakfast, or lunch, and going long periods without eating, but have high body fat levels. Want to know why their body fat is still so high?

If you go a really long period without eating, what usually happens to your hunger? You get RAVENOUSLY hungry, right? Then what do you do when you do finally sit down to eat? You eat like Miss Piggy at a buffet! You consume everything that's not nailed down. You consume tons and tons of calories, which usually ends up with you eating MORE than your calorie limits. This usually ends up with you over-consuming like crazy and then you store fat because you ate too many calories. You see, it wasn't "starvation mode," but the lack of planning, preparation, and focus that led to BINGE mode. They are just simply OVEREATING when they do eat and usually of all the wrong foods, too.

So they starved all day, possibly burning muscle, which led to them getting ravenously hungry and BINGEING at night.

They are consistently consuming tons of calories leading to a surplus and fat gain. Or they ate an amount equivalent to what they burned, so they lose NOTHING. No deficit, no loss. Period!

But yet they claim "I never eat. I need to eat more often. I'm not eating enough." BULLSHIT!

Yeah, these same people tend to often forget to mention their nightly binge or the six Starbucks calorie-packed sugar bombs or the 8 sodas they inhale during the day. But its starvation mode, right? STFU!

It's NOT your body that's not responding. Your body is doing exactly what you FORCE it to do. You either force it to store fat or your force it to get shredded. I've found that those that are the heaviest play the biggest victims and are the biggest liars living in denial about how they eat. They mindlessly consume thousands of excess calories from processed foods and don't even blink.

So if you have been this person in the past or are this complainer right now, now you know why. So quit playing a little bitch victim and FIX it. Dial in your macros, track food accurately, create a deficit, do it consistently, and you will get SHREDDED!

Everything adds up

"You can live in the gym, but if you don't get your nutrition dialed in, you're wasting your time."
-Unknown

Another issue most people do that affects the speed of their results is adding small doses of calories each meal. This adds up to A LOT by the end of a day. Everything you consume has calories, even most of those so-called zero-calorie products. If a product has less than 5 calories per serving, they can legally claim zero calories. EVERYTHING except water has calories. So everything you eat adds up – every bite, every handful, every taste, every sauce, every oil you cook with – everything you eat has calories. It adds up very, very quickly. How? Let's give you an example.

Joe is supposed to be eating 2,200 calories a day to get shredded (creating a deficit) and he burns about 3,000 (TDEE) a day on the days he trains. He has all his meals planned and measured out perfectly, packed all his meals, and are perfectly at 2,200 calories. But Joe didn't account for the little things:

- Joe added coffee creamer to his coffee twice, which he didn't account for.   +160 calories (which is sugar, creating more cravings later)
- Joe added marinara sauce to his meals, which he didn't account for. +90 Calories
- Joe took a bite of his coworker's pizza during lunch. +90 calories
- Joe also cooked his food in coconut oil but he didn't track it. +120 calories.
- Joe was craving more after his last meal, had handful of nuts. +450 calories
- Prepped food was 2,200 calories.

90 + 120 + 450 = 3,110 total calories for the day.

Joe actually got fatter today.

Yet tomorrow he will be the first one to say "I don't know what's going on! I'm eating right and work out but I keep getting fat! I think I have a slow metabolism. It's my genes. I think I have thyroid issue. I think I have a fat gene. I just can't lose any weight."

Joe, STFU! You're full of shit and all your little undisciplined, unaccounted choices added up to a calorie SURPLUS! This is a TYPICAL American. This is probably YOU. This example here is 99% of gym goers today, which is one of the reasons why they all look just as fat this year as they did LAST year, or maybe even a little fatter. Now you know why. If this is you, IT STOPS NOW. EVERYTHING COUNTS!

Everything adds up, and the more you eat, the less fat you're going to burn. Eat too much and you don't lose an ounce. Eat more than you burn and you gain body fat. So obsessively weigh your portions and track your intake, so you STAY in a deficit. Once your calories and macros have been met, you're DONE. Drink water and take your ass to bed. How many days a week should your macros be on point? All seven days!

Now let's discuss a few rules of nutrition

I have found that even though I take the time to write up personalized meal plans for my online and in-person clients, they tend to just always make their own. They just follow the shredder system.

When it comes to eating, remember that it's all about the total calories and macros for the day. We have to create a deficit and make smart choices, but there is a system of doing things. Implement a systematic way of eating that you want to make your new permanent habit.

Work the system and you get shredded.

Shredder System Of Eating

Want to learn the basic rules to follow so you can get shredded?

1. PVF: Protein and Veggies First!

What's the number one rule when it comes to eating? What's the staple for all of your meals? PVF! We already discussed this but I want to reiterate it so it sinks in. The simple rule of thumb to keeping your calories and macros in check is to ALWAYS eat protein and veggies first. This keeps you blood sugar levels in check, triggers the release of certain hormones, keeps your energy levels steady, keeps you feeling fuller, and keeps you from overeating and from having cravings.

Now your calorie requirements vary by a few hundred depending on your height, weight, and activity. But generally the average man needs 2100-2500 calories per day to burn fat. The shorter and lighter you are, the less you need; the taller you are, or more muscular you are, the more you can have.

The simple rule of **PVF** will naturally make you eat less calories because of the hormonal response and the time it takes to digest, so don't be surprised if you can't eat all your meals at first. As your body gets used to eating these foods consistently, it will feel more normal.

2. Track it BEFORE you eat it.

What's the best way to prevent making mistakes so your macros are on point seven days a week? Weigh and track your food on your MyFitnessPal app BEFORE you eat. Always do this so you are accurate and don't make mistakes and overeat.

If you track AFTER you eat, you are more than likely going to end up overeating and then going, "OOPS!" No oopsies. Track first before you eat anything.

You may find that towards the end of the day, that you may need a lot more fats or need more protein because you are behind, so your meal will have to adjust for that. Typically, most people's carbs are usually done earlier. So your last meal, or meals will have to be modified to hit your macros. It's okay to be lower on carbs, but always make sure you hit your protein and fat requirements. It's also okay to have just fats or just protein in your last meal if that's what you need more of.

These are priority. As matter of fact, if carbs are lower, eat MORE protein or fats to get your calories closer to the recommended calorie limit.

3. Cook food in bulk.

What's the easy way to prepare foods? Cook in bulk. Cook up 5-10 pounds of protein, boil and peel two dozen eggs, bake some sweet potatoes, or cook up some quinoa, all in bulk. This makes your preparation a cinch. Always have food made in bulk. If you do this right, you really only need to cook two to three times a week.

4. Plan ahead.

What do you need to do each night to prep for the next day? Pack food every night for the following day. Cook, weigh, pack, and even track your meals each night for the next day. You know how long you are going to be gone from home for work and errands, so bring enough food to last.

If you go unprepared, you STARVE until you get home. Not having food is not an excuse to eat crap, eat out, or make poor choices. So if you fail to plan ahead, punish yourself and starve until you get home. You're not going to die. Starving for a short period is better than overeating from going out to eat. Planning gets easier as it becomes a habit.

5. Macros seven days a week.

What do you need to do seven days a week? Hit your macros! The example meal plans are set up to simplify nutrition, but you will probably make your own. This is fine as long as you follow the rules of the Shredder System to hit your macros seven days a week, every week.

6. Deficit Days 6-13

What do we have to create to burn fat? A calorie deficit! How many days do we stay in a deficit? There are many ways of doing this, but for simplicity purposes of this program, we are going to split this into two categories: the leaner group, the heavier group. The leaner group deficits for six days straight, while the heavier group deficits for 13 days straight.

What differentiates them?

If you are leaner, meaning near single-digit body fat percentage or are slightly higher but you are very active and athletic, you fall into the leaner category. You are going to stay in a deficit for six days straight. If you are heavier, you go for 13 days of deficit.

If you are somewhere in the middle, just start with the 13 days. Being that the average guy in America is 196 lb., I'm sure your body fat is higher than you think it is. As you get leaner and into single-digit body fat, then you move to six days of deficit.

Stay in a deficit consistently to consistently burn fat. Then on that seventh/fourteenth day, what do you do? You do what's known as a Refeed Day.

#7. Refeed to burn more fat.

"Refeed is taking one step back, but two steps forward."
–Josef Rakich

<u>Note</u>: **YOU MUST train on this day. You cannot do a high calorie day on a day off. No train, no refeed.**

What is a refeed? A refeed is basically a day where you REFEED your body by increasing your carb intake, which increases your calories to promote certain fat-burning hormones and keep your body melting fat. We do this because if you stay in a deficit too long, your body will start to feel threatened and possibly start to burn muscle for energy, eliminating muscle to become more efficient, and reducing the amount of body fat it is using for energy. By refeeding every one to two weeks, it basically it refeeds your body to make it feel like it's not starving, so it continues to burn fat.

Pick a specific day (Saturday or Sunday is a typical choice) and stick to it. This day, just eat more CARBS: more fruit, more oats, quinoa, etc. But just like any other day, the Shredder Rules apply, especially the PVF rule and staying UNDER your calorie limit.

Calorie limits vary, from 2,800-4,500 depending on your height, weight, activity levels, etc. I'd recommend starting on the lower end, then watching your body to see if you can add more and get away with it. If you feel or look fatter after, reduce calories. If you're okay, stay the same or add 100-200 calories more next time.

The rule of thumb is to burn 1,000+ calories on this day. When we get into the training, you'll understand how to find out how much you're burning.

Refeed Example:

So for Average Joe, this day he would eat 3,000 calories and about 350 g of those calories would be from carbs. Just follow the PVF (protein and veggies first) rule, then add more carbs to your meals. Make sure it is weighed, tracked, and accounted for so that you do NOT go over your limit. Also make sure you train HARD that day.

Meal #1: PVF and 60g carbs (fruit, brown rice, quinoa, etc.)
Meal #2: PVF and 60g carbs (fruit, brown rice, quinoa, etc.)
Meal #3: PVF and 60g carbs (fruit, brown rice, quinoa, etc.)
Meal #4: PVF and 60g carbs (fruit, brown rice, quinoa, etc.)
Meal #5: PVF and 60g carbs (fruit, brown rice, quinoa, etc.)

The most important element is staying under your refeed day calorie limit. Remember, it doesn't matter if you do this in three meals or in five. You will be pretty full on this day. Once your calories are met, you're done. Drink water and get to bed. You will feel like Superman in your next workout. Then it's back on track and eating in deficit for another 6-13 days.

That is the simplified explanation of how you do a refeed day. Your nutrition plan examples have examples of how to do this. Pretty easy, huh? Good. Now let's move on to some other key elements to your fat burning.

Water is one of the secrets to fat loss

"Water is the driving force of all nature."
–Leonardo Da Vinci

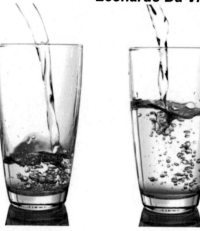
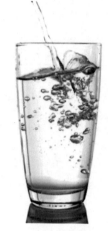

The human body is made up of about 70% water, our muscles consist of about 80% water, your blood is 90% water, and your liver is 95% water. Being adequately hydrated is a crucial element to getting shredded and feeling great. We are losing fluids all day long, with every breath and trip to the bathroom, so water has to be replenished ALL day long. Most people are chronically dehydrated and aren't even aware of it. As a matter of fact, each morning when you wake up, you are dehydrated from the start because you haven't had in fluids in five to eight hours. This is WHY you feel so groggy in the morning.

Being dehydrated has a whole host of issues associated with it. From poor health, altered body temperature control, reduced motivation, fatigue, make training feel very difficult mentally and physically, and causing you to be moody. This is also the number one reason you drag ass when the alarm clock goes off each morning.

Being dehydrated just 1-3% completely impairs your brain function, leading to poor memory, poor concentration, and even frequent headaches. Being dehydrated also causes constipation. Yes, you need water to drop the kids off, too.

Dehydration also makes you look PUFFY. When your body doesn't get enough water, it holds onto what it has. Being dehydrated will make your body retain water as a survival mechanism, which will make you look like the Stay Puff Marshmallow Man. Usually, you can really see this in people's faces.

Dehydration leads to aches and pains. It is why you suddenly lose energy or motivation to train during workouts, or even the reason why you couldn't muster the energy to start. Dehydration is also why you feel dips in energy at the office, during the day. You are dehydrated!

Dehydration can also trigger carb cravings. So if you feel cravings for carbs coming on or even hunger for no reason, that could be a sign you're behind on your water intake. Slam 40 ounces of water and watch the cravings disappear.

Some studies say that being dehydrated 3-5% can decrease your muscle strength by up to 30%. Imagine how crappy your training is going to be if you're only able to put in 70% of your capability. So needless to say, being adequately hydrated is very important and a requirement to burning fat and getting shredded.

"Water is the MOST important nutrient in the body."
-Dr. Michael Colgan, Sports Nutritionist

Water is essential to the fat burning process. Not only do you need it for health, you NEED it to burn fat. One of the important functions of your kidneys is to eliminate toxic waste products from your body through urine. When you're dehydrated, the body instinctively retains whatever water it does have to survive. When this happens waste products are not flushed out and they build up in your system.

At this point, the liver starts to help out with the work. One of the main organs responsible for fat burning is your liver, but when the kidneys aren't functioning properly to eliminate toxins, the liver has to come to the rescue and help out. If your liver is busy eliminating toxins, that means it has less focus to burn body fat for you.

"Drinking water is like taking a shower on the inside."
-Unknown

So as you can see, keeping the body adequately hydrated is extremely important to your success in getting shredded. Drinking lots of water does NOT make you retain water; being DEHYDRATED does. For some reason, people think that their "water retention" comes from drinking water. Nope, quite the opposite. For the most part, any time you have had that feeling of water retention, you more than likely just recently ate A LOT of processed foods or high sodium foods. However, you're still primarily retaining because you haven't consumed enough water.

"Hydrate, feel GREAT!"
–Unknown

Benefits of proper hydration

- Studies have shown that drinking water can increase your metabolism and help you burn up to an extra 96 calories per day. It doesn't sound like much but that's almost an extra pound of fat burned in just 35 days from just sipping on some water.
- Water makes you a more efficient fat burner. Remember the facts about the liver I just mentioned. The liver is what removes toxins from the body, stores fat-soluble vitamins, and is responsible for breaking down fatty acids and transporting them to the blood to be metabolized. We want to make sure it is working at 100%! This is done by HYDRATING!
- Water reduces water retention and will actually make you look LEANER and your muscles FULLER, which means you will look BETTER.
- Water improves your mood and makes you feel happier. Any time you feel cranky or moody for no reason, that's a sign you're dehydrated, so drink up!
- Water increases your energy. Feeling tired is a sign of dehydration and filling up on water can quickly put the pep back into your mental step within the hour.
- Water keeps your joints lubricated and hydrated. Cartilage is 85% water, so keeping this protective material hydrated and healthy is a must so that your joints feel good.
- Water makes you eat less. When adequately hydrated, you feel more satiety throughout the day, meaning you will naturally eat less.
- Water aids in the detoxification process. It also transports nutrients, aids digestion, and regulates body temperature.

- Water improves your skin and boosts immune system.
- Water improves your performance. This is one of the areas that being adequately hydrated is crucial: your performance. When you are adequately hydrated ,you can train hard, train more intense, pump out more reps, work out longer, lift heavier, which ultimately means MORE results for you.

Besides having your macros on point, your water intake is also a very important element you MUST also have on point.

How much water?

I'm sure you've heard the old saying of "Drink 8 to 10 8-ouce glasses a day." Well, its BS. There's no frickin' way this would be an adequate amount to adequately hydrate you with the lifestyle WE live. If you are sedentary and sitting on your ass all day, not working out, and not moving, then sure, that may be sufficient. But this is YOU, you are a Shredded Exec, you are going to be training like a BEAST daily. Which means you are going to need A LOT more water to be able to function and perform the way that is required to get shredded.

Now the amount is truly dependent on your size, activity, and the amount you sweat but generally you need to consume 1.5 to three gallons PER DAY. Yes, you read that right. The bigger you are and the more you sweat, the more you need. I recommend at LEAST 1 ounce of water per pound of bodyweight. Just an FYI: 128 ounces equals 1 gallon, which for most of you will be over 1.5 gallons or per day.

Most of you don't drink anywhere near this much, so most of you don't even get the old-school 8 to 10 8-ounce glasses per day. This is WHY you're not looking or performing at the levels you are capable of. I'm right, I know. It is very common for Americans to be chronically dehydrated.

Quick hydration test

Want to know the trick to see how hydrated you are? Think about the frequency of your pee. When was the last time you peed? What color was it? Do you know how often you should be peeing to be considered accurately hydrated?

In my opinion, if you are hydrated, you should be peeing every 15 to 30 minutes and it would be clear or almost clear. If you aren't peeing that often or your pee looks like apple juice, you are severely dehydrated and everything within your body is suffering tremendously. Your energy sucks, your mood sucks, your performance in the gym is going to suck, and you look puffy. So what do you need to do right now? Hydrate! It's time to step your game up and get your hydration and your results up!

Personally, I'm about 5'6" and around 150 pounds – and I drink over 3.5 gallons per day. Anything less than that and I feel like shit. Obviously, I've worked my way up to this, and am very active. But when you are hydrated, you will FEEL the difference and you will feel awesome!

Want to know the hack to easily hydrate?

The hydration hack

This is very simple: keep two to three full gallons of water with you DAILY. Your goal is to drink 1.5 to three gallons, depending on your needs. I would refill or buy new ones daily and put them your vehicle each night so you are ready for the next day.

For instance, let's say your goal is to drink two gallons per day. Each night, you would fill or buy two gallons of water, and put them in your vehicle for the next day. Each day, finish those two containers. I know it sounds like common sense, but you wouldn't believe how many people try to keep track of actual glasses or small water bottles. This often leads to them forgetting how many glasses or bottles they have consumed and often leaves them dehydrated. Therefore, utilize at least two gallon jugs daily.

How to drink faster

Drinking straight out of a gallon jug is rather awkward, especially if you are in public or an office, which also leads to you drinking it slower. Another hack to increase water consumption quickly, is to keep a big protein shaker cup with you at all times. Pour the water from your gallon into this cup and chug it. Always keep this cup full. Do this once or twice an hour. Before you know it, your water intake is sufficient and you are looking and feeling awesome!

I personally use this exact same process. I have two gallon jugs that I refill every day and carry them around in my truck. (I also have a water filter on my home water system.) This is the easiest way to keep track and measure how much you have consumed. My goal is to drink the first two gallons before 12:00 p.m. As long as I am on pace for that, my workouts and energy levels are at their best. Then I just drink the other 1.5 gallons throughout the rest of the day.

When you start to hydrate adequately, you will feel the difference literally within the hour because you will have more energy, be in a better mood, happier, and you'll kick ass in your training. This will be noticeable, especially after just a day or two.

Add salt!

Along with increasing your water intake, we also need to increase your salt intake. Wait, what? Yep, you read that right.

Thanks to another misguided government mistake, we have been led to believe that salt is dangerous and unhealthy, kind of like how saturated fat was demonized. They believed it increased blood pressure and was a risk factor for heart disease and stroke. Once again, it wasn't the salt that is causing the issue, it was processed foods.

Due to today's high processed foods diets, people get more than enough salt. But with your new healthy whole-food diet, you're going to need to ADD salt to your day. This is not the terrible table salt, I'm talking about. Instead, I'm speaking of pink Himalayan salt that is full of trace minerals.

So with the increase of your water intake and the elimination of your processed foods, you need to make sure you get enough salt. Salt is actually GOOD for you if you use it wisely. It will actually help you train harder, lift more, improve your cellular functions, cellular communication, make your muscles hold more water and look fuller, increase vascularity, and pump muscle.

Salt is rich in minerals, with some studies showing it contains 84 minerals, electrolytes, and elements. It is an essential nutrient that our bodies require for transporting nutrients into and out of our cells, regulating blood pressure, exchanging ions, and so much more. Simply put, getting adequate salt in your diet will help make you a BEAST in training and in the mirror. Adding salt to water can make you look and perform like a superhero.

So feel free to add salt to your food. Just make sure you utilize the beneficial ones like pink Himalayan or sea salt, because these have trace minerals. I personally prefer Himalayan.

How to consume it

Note: Do not add this to your daily gallon jugs as it is not as effective as doing it the way I'm about to recommend.

One of the best ways to make sure you have an awesome workout is to make sure you start your day with some Superhero Water. This is one of MY personal creations, a secret that only my clients and workout partners know about. But because you are now part of my crew, I'm going to share this with you.

There is a little concoction I created that works like a charm and turns you into an unstoppable animal in your workouts. It makes you able to sustain your intensity during our INSANE trainings. Like I just mentioned, salt used properly is actually BENEFICIAL to the body and important for your diet. Our bodies rely on electrolytes, including salt to help carry out electrical impulses that control many of our bodily functions. Salt is important to the nerves as it stimulates muscle contractions. Salt also plays a primary role in the processes of digestion and absorption. Sodium deficiency is very dangerous. So this is how we make sure you are getting an adequate amount.

Here's the secret recipe:

Superhero hydration. (2-3x per day. Upon waking, before training, after training)
- ½ tsp. salt (Himalayan or sea salt)
- 20 oz. water (protein shake cup)

As soon as you wake up(morning person hack remember), eat some protein and down this Superhero Water. Then drink another 20 ounces water. This means you need to drink 40 ounces right off the bat as soon as you get up. Yes, you may be full, but so what? Stop being a 'lil bitch and man up.

This is perfect if you train early morning. Get up, eat, Superhero hydrate, go train like a beast, and then go be the boss of your day. If you train later in the day, do another Superhero water right before training. You need to Superhero hydrate upon waking, and/or before and after training.

Make sure you carry a full gallon of regular water with you to the gym and drink in between sets. If you feel your energy levels dip at all during training, that's a sign you NEED more water or you need salt if you have been training hard or long. Keep a container of salt and a teaspoon in your gym bag.

During my workouts, I personally carry my protein shaker cup and a gallon, and make sure to down a shaker cup full of water around every 15-20 minutes. Get in the habit of doing this and you will be able to train harder, longer. This means faster results and more shreds for you.

Always make sure you do a serving of salt post-workout as well. This will speed your body's ability to recover and make you feel GOOD. If you ever feel like crap, especially after training, it's because you're either dehydrated, or salt depleted. Always make sure you get sufficient water and salt daily. This is why I recommend you always do the Superhero Water before and after training as a minimum.

We are all different, so this is something you can play with adding more. As your program progresses, you may find you need more salt added to your diet daily. That's okay. Go for it! Just make sure you are sweating and consuming a lot of water.

Okay, so we talked about the importance of hydration and I gave you my secret concoction of Superhero hydration. Now, let's briefly talk supplements.

Supplements

Would you like to know which supplements are going to help you melt fat? Would you like to know which supplements are going to make you build more muscle?

Well, too bad. You have been duped by today's marketing copywriters, because 99.999999% of supplements are pure crap. Most supplements you see in the magazines, on TV, and on store shelves are completely useless and unnecessary. Supplements are BIG business and Americans spend nearly $35 Billion on diets and weight loss products. There are a thousand different manufacturers, 20,000 different products consumed by over 100 million people, and 99.9999999% of it is bullshit. These companies will tell you anything they think you want to hear so they can have a piece of that $35 Billion.

So before you go investing in all kinds of products that are going to help you "build muscle, burn fat, get shredded, and get ripped," know that most magazines OWN supplement companies. Did you ever notice how there's always a supplement recommendation tied to those tips they give? You read the article talking about an incredible training program or way of burning fat and then somewhere tied into the article, there is a promotion of some supplement. Ever notice that?

Go pick up a magazine or read an article from a well-established company. You will see it now. These prints make it appear more credible to consumers mentally, but I'll tell you now that MOST supplements are complete bullshit. There's no magic in protein powders, no magic in fat burners, and no magic creatine. Can they help? Maybe, but you're talking by like 1%.

Your results aren't going to come from a bottle, pill or powder. They are going to come from GOOD nutrition, eating REAL food, getting your macros on point seven days a week, and by consistently training intensely. Doing these things consistently over TIME leads to getting shredded, not by taking pills. Not by some highly processed protein powder that is truly a low-quality form of protein. What you want requires REAL food, REAL nutrients, and REAL sweat.

Another thing you need to know too is that the models representing these products did NOT get their physiques from these products. They were signed AFTER they already had the physique and they attained that physique through YEARS and YEARS of hard work and good NUTRITION. Then they got popular, got noticed by a supplement company, and the company signed them to represent their product so they can sell even more products.

It's like Michael Jordan or Tiger Woods being signed by Nike. Did Nike make these athletes? Fuvk no! They spent decades training, learning, improving, and mastering their craft to become one of the best athletes ever, and THEN they got the endorsements. This is exactly how these athletes got their physiques: by years and years of hard work.

Notice what I just said about how these guys earned their physiques? Years and years of HARD work and nutrition. NOT from some stupid pill, powder, or protein shake.

On another note, most of these models (I'd estimate 99%) did supplement their training to obtain these physiques, but it wasn't a protein shake that got them jacked, and it wasn't a fat burner that got them shredded. Instead, it came in the form of a performance enhancing drug. Most of the fitness models and bodybuilders you see, are NOT natural. Yep, not natural and not truly earned, in my opinion. They have been using drugs for YEARS. They are where they are because of the DRUGS.

Unless they compete in a stringent drug testing federation and have 10-20 years under their belt, don't believe a word they say. What works for a juicehead will not work the same for you. I firmly believe that it's their lives. They can do what they want, but just know they are NOT natural. Steroids did it, not the protein powder. Diuretics, thyroid meds, and other drugs I don't even know about or understand got them shredded, not the fat burners.

Take away the drugs and these guys would instantly lose 50-75% of their gains instantly! So what's really creating those results? You guessed it: drugs. And they KNOW it too, which is why you'll rarely ever see any of them off of the drugs until they DIE or retire.

I'm anti-drugs. If you choose to take that route, that's your choice. You know the risks (death, enlarged organs, heart attacks are most common, kidney failure, bitch tits, small testicles, acne, rages, depression, etc.). Your body, your life. What I'm teaching can be accomplished 100% naturally through implementing the things I share in this book. I'm teaching you to achieve this the RIGHT way. Earn it and keep it!

DON'T BE A SUCKER for supplements. Your answer to getting shredded will ONLY come from good nutrition and training done consistently over time.

On the other side of this – the health side – the great majority of supplements (vitamins and minerals), an estimated 95% of them are actually manufactured by Big Pharma. Yup, you read that right. Drug companies are the primary manufacturer of most of the supplements you see on the shelves. This means they are synthetic, so synthetic vitamins and minerals do not work optimally, if at all, in the body. As a matter of fact, some studies show they are actually harmful.

Check your labels

Always read labels and ingredients list. Vitamins and minerals that are in true form will have some form of vegetable, fruit, etc. in the ingredient list. If you see anything that ends with -ite, -ate, or -ide, it is synthetic, so trash it.

For instance, if you see chloride, hydrochloride, acetate, bitartrate, gluconate, stearate, succinate, or nitrate, these are synthetics. If there are any letters in front of the name like *dl* or *L,* these are synthetics. A very common one is magnesium stearate. This is junk.

A true vitamin or mineral will have a FOOD source in the ingredients list. For instance, magnesium would have spinach or a rice bran in the ingredients list because it comes from a food source. Vitamin C would have acerola cherry powder in the ingredients list. If you can see the actual name of a vitamin or mineral in the ingredients list, it's almost a guarantee that it is fake. Look for food in the ingredients list and pure names of vitamins and minerals, like magnesium by itself.

Now that we have cleared up the fake, let's talk about some supplements that I DO recommend that will have a dramatic effect on your training, performance, mentality, and which will lead to better results.

Multivitamins and minerals

In order for your body to feel, perform, look its absolute best, you have to be replenishing the raw materials that it needs to FUNCTION and perform its best. This comes from Vitamins and minerals. Now that your diet is going to be healthier, you will be getting a lot more of these nutrients naturally. But there are TONS you may not be getting because you don't eat certain foods. I have found most people tend to stick to the same core foods – even me.

There are thousands of nutrients you are missing out on that these other foods provide. You are also going to be training very intensely, so your micronutrient needs are going to be very high because you are going to lose them on a daily basis, so they must be replenished.

Micronutrients by definition are essential nutrients, such as a mineral or vitamin that is required for the proper growth and metabolism of an organism. Along with getting your macros (proteins, carbs, and fats), you also need your micros (vitamins and minerals). Think of your macros as providing energy and building materials, while the micros are different components that provide the "workers" to make the body function.

Nutrient deficiencies are linked to EVERY disease known to man. Being depleted of any of the essential micros is like opening the door for disease. It also cannot perform, sleep, recover, train, or get adequate energy production. Constantly replenishing and flooding your system with nutrients is key to optimal health and aesthetics.

Since most people are creatures of habit and tend to eat the same foods daily, your diet will be missing a lot of nutrients that could benefit it. So to close that gap, we supplement with a high-quality multivitamin and multimineral. Remember, most supplements on the market are synthetic crap, and as of today, one of the ONLY brands that I have found that is high-quality and comes straight from the farm to a capsule or tablet is the brand called Mega Food. There may be more companies out there, but so far Mega Food brand is my go to company for micros.

Out of all the micros, there is one mineral that I feel is one of the MOST important, that magic mineral is Magnesium. The great fitness gurus like Charles Poliquin, Paul Chek, and physicians like Dr. Mercola and Dr. Hyman would agree that magnesium is the most important. It is also the one that most people are extremely deficient in, as an estimated 80% of Americans already are.

We talked about this one a little bit in the chapter about how to become a morning person, but there's more to this magic mineral.

Being deficient in magnesium can trigger tons of medical conditions, from anxiety and panic attacks, asthma, blood clots, bowel diseases, depression, hypertension, insomnia kidney disease, liver disease, migraines, fibromyalgia, cramps, muscle pain, nerve problems, PMS and infertility, osteoporosis, tooth decay, numbness and tingling, muscle spasms and cramps, seizures, personality changes, abnormal heart rhythms, coronary spasms, nausea, fatigue, headache, weakness, poor immunity, ADD and ADHD like behaviors, and low testosterone.

It is literally NECESSARY for over 300+ biochemical reactions in the body. Magnesium is involved in virtually every metabolic process in the body. From heart health, muscle contractions, hormone production (testosterone and growth hormone), sleep, recovery, digestion, memory, energy production, improving strength, decreasing inflammation, and stronger bones, all of which are integral parts of getting the BEST results, developing muscle, and getting SHREDDED.

I personally didn't start supplementing this until a couple of years ago, and I'm telling you now, it is a NIGHT and DAY difference on how you train, sleep, lift, and how much more of a beast this little mineral makes you. If there is ONE magic supplement, MAGNESIUM is it. Which is why I am telling you to make it part of your daily intake.

Like I said, the only brand I currently recommend is Mega Food brand. You can find it online, or at most health food stores. Take 4-6 tablets before bed as well. You will immediately notice the improvements in your quality of sleep. You will sleep deep and wake up refreshed. Along with your multivitamin, keep this bottle by your bedside on your night stand and take it about 30-60 minutes before bed.

Expect to have crazy, vivid dreams. You are going to sleep very fully and have plenty of REM sleep, so your dreams are going to be intense. I'm already laughing inside thinking about the look on your face you're going to have in the mornings after you wake up with a "WTF!!?" look on your face from your dreams.

Omega 3

We discussed this one earlier in this book, but I wanted to mention this to make sure you remember and focus on getting an adequate amount. We get our best Omega 3 from fish oil or Krill oil. If you're taking fish oil, you will need 10-15 capsules per day. If you're doing Krill oil, a good rule of thumb is 5-10 capsules per day. These are the MOST important fats in my opinion and are complete game changers. Make sure you supplement these into your diet.

Fish oil liquid, take 2-3 tsp. a day, and just take all at once.

Getting Omega 3 is crucial to your overall health, and performance, which directly affects your results and aesthetics, so supplement wisely!

Vitamin D3

Another common vitamin deficiency that is also linked to most diseases is vitamin D. Low Vitamin D is related to cancer, depression, Alzheimer's, diabetes, all the major diseases. But this one is a cool one because you can manufacture it yourself, with your own body. But many people are missing the key ingredient to produce it. It is also more utilized as a hormone within the body.

"It regulates more genes and bodily functions than any other hormone yet discovered."
–Dr. Mercola

There have been numerous studies done on this vitamin over the past recent years, it is shown that having adequate Vitamin D levels is a requirement for optimal health and performance. Want to know what that one ingredient you need to produce Vitamin D is?

SUNLIGHT!

Sunlight on your skin makes your body produce Vitamin D. When your body has an adequate amount of Vitamin D, it improves your immune system, strengthens bones, increases production of leptin, the hormone that makes you feel full, so you naturally eat less. Fat cells slow their efforts to make or store fat, so you will burn more fat.

You will also reduce the production of cortisol, the stress hormone that causes belly fat. Vitamin D also activates genes and cells signaling chemicals that are responsible for muscle growth, strength, and performance. Vitamin D is also important for the development of testosterone. Vital for testosterone production so always get your D.

Do you see now why this is a critical vitamin to be sufficient in? Good. So do your best to get 15-20 minutes of sunlight on your skin three to seven days per week to produce it. If you cannot get enough sun, supplement Vitamin D3 around 5,000+ IU minimum per day. Sunlight is best because you will produce much more than what you get from supplements.

Now that we have talked about the healthy necessities, let's discuss the supplements that will give you that extra umph to push harder in training: pre-workouts.

Pre-workouts

As you have seen throughout this entire book, I am a huge believer in natural, nature-made, foods, and products to develop a shredded physique. There is one exception to this, and that exception is a pre-workout supplement.

This is the only thing that is not natural that I would recommend ever putting in your body. And even then, you don't have to take this; it is just an option. You can do cleaner, healthier forms, like green tea, a double shot of black coffee, or caffeine pills. I do these from time to time as well.

The pre-workouts I am speaking about are the ones made by supplement companies, and there are literally HUNDREDS on the market today. Personally, I highly recommend you DO take some form of a stimulant for a pre-workout prior to daily training. The real and only reason is because it is going to make you train HARDER. The harder you train, the more results you develop, plain and simple.

I have tried them all and they all have slightly different effects on people. My recommendation is to try one and keep testing new ones to see which kind works best for you.

Go to www.bodybuilding.com and take your pick. Read nutrition labels and make sure it is not a carb drink. Know that most pre-workouts contain sucralose (Splenda) as a sweetener. Sucralose is very damaging to your gut bacteria, which is why the smaller the dose, the better. This is also why you need to supplement with probiotics as well. Pre-workouts are the ONLY unnatural product that is allowed. But like I said, you can choose cleaner options. It is your choice. But take something so that way, you can work your ass off. Make sure your diet, sodium, and water are on point as well.

Now that we have discussed pre-workouts, let's talk probiotics.

Probiotics

Your gut is known as your second brain, also known as the enteric nervous system. It is called the second brain because while it communicates with the brain, it also has the ability to act independently and influence your behavior. There are about 400-600 million neurons (nerve cells are electrically excitable cells that processes and transmit information through electrical and chemical signals).

You are not conscious of your gut thinking, but the system produces about 95% of the serotonin and 50% of the dopamine found in your body. It is the home of 80% of your immune system. One of the reasons why your gut has so much influence on your health has to do with the 100 TRILLION bacteria that line your intestinal tract. That's about three pounds worth of bacteria in your gut – some good, some not so good. This extremely complex living system is designed to protect your body from outside invaders.

With today's SAD (standard American diet), most people's second brain is truly out of balance and compromised. Processed foods (sugar, flour, processed oils, and dairy) cause gaps (leaky gut) in the intestinal lining, allowing bad bugs and undigested food particles into the bloodstream, leading to systemic inflammation. These same foods FEED the fungus and bad bacteria that live in our guts, leading to them growing exponentially. This further leads to frequent sickness, bloating, gas, skin disorders, allergies, chronic disease, autoimmune diseases, joint and muscle pain, and a host of other illnesses.

Why does this matter? The healthier your gut, the healthier you are, the better you will feel, the better you will train, the better you absorb nutrients, the better your results, the better you look, and the happier you are. I am all about getting you shredded, but I want you shredded AND healthy.

So along with feeding your body a diet high in nutritious food, you should also take a good quality probiotic. These are your GOOD bacteria that are responsible for your health and optimal performance. The good bacteria in your gut also feed off of fiber, so eating more veggies will help shift your microbiome (bacteria) into one that is correlated with leanness.

So avoid antibiotics and TAKE probiotics. Avoid processed foods (sugar, flour, manmade foods) and eat plenty of veggies with healthy sources of protein. One of the other reasons why magnesium and Omega 3s are so important is also because of the positive effect they have on your gut. They all work together to benefit your overall health and performance.

These are the only supplements that I recommend. Did you notice how I didn't mention protein powders or fat burners? I didn't mention carnitine, CLA, creatine, or anything else. Want to know why? Because you don't NEED them! That's how brainwashed you have become from all the magazines and articles written by supplement companies.

Your results come from number one, nutrition (eating REAL foods with lots of nutrients), and secondly, intense training done consistently. These two done over time equal a shredded physique. No magic, just purely done the RIGHT way for optimal health and shredded wealth.

Results come from real food, heavy weight training, and strategic nutrition are BETTER than supplements and better than drugs, because there are no side effects and the results are PERMANENT (as long as you keep training and eating right).

So stop looking for a quick fix and stop looking for a magic pill, because it doesn't exist. (Although magnesium, salt, and Omega 3s are pretty badass). The only way you're going to get this shredded body and stay there is by making PERMANENT lifestyle changes. Lifting hard, and hitting your macros with real foods is a must to achieve success. You do this because this is WHO you are, and WHAT you do.

That sums up nutrition. Let's move on to how to socialize.

Review:

1. What is your BMR?
2. What is your TDEE?
3. What is getting shredded?
4. How do you make the body burn fat to get shredded?
5. What makes the body store fat?
6. "No____, no loss. Period.
7. What percentage of your results is based off of your nutrition?
8. What does PVF stand for?
9. When do you track your food?
10. Cook food in ____ for easy prep.
11. How many days a week do you need to hit your macros?
12. How many days do you need to deficit? How often refeed?
13. Why do we refeed?
14. How many calories do you need to burn on refeed day?
15. How much water should you be drinking a day?
16. What is Superhero Water?
17. When should you drink Superhero Water?
18. What is the magic mineral? How many per night?
19. What is the best fat?
20. What vitamin is considered a hormone?
21. What is a cleaner version of pre-workout?
22. What is considered your second brain? What should you supplement it with?

[8]
Lifestyle

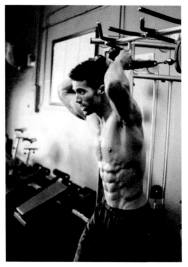

-Jake Barrena (My buddy and business partner)

Getting shredded is a lifestyle and in this chapter I am going to give you a few tricks on how expedite your success, how to live, how to deal with people, how to socialize, how to eat out, how to drink, and how to prep for holidays.

First, let's talk about one of the success hacks that you probably already know when it comes to business and finances, but this is especially crucial when it comes to you getting shredded.

What do you think is the biggest determining factor of your level of success in life?

Your parents? Your education?

According to studies done by Harvard, the biggest determining factor to the level of success you achieve in life is your PEER group. Yep, not your parents or education, but the people you choose to be around, the people you associate with are the biggest determining factor of the level of success you achieve in life.

"You are the average of the five people you spend the most time with."
-Jim Rohn

So what does that mean? This means, take the average income, physique, mindset, relationship status, of the people you spend the most time with, that is your future.

Take the average body, attitude, and lifestyle habits of the people you spend your time with, that's your future body, future attitude, and future lifestyle.

So, if you...

Hang out with five idiots, you become the sixth.

Hang out with five overweight people, you become the sixth.

Who you spend time with influences the person you will eventually become. The type of people you interact with influences the level you operate in, the subject matter you engage in, the mindset, the way of thinking, the behaviors, the actions you take, and even the way you speak.

Think about it, I'm sure you have unfit and overweight friends right now. What do they like to do? What does their entire life revolve around? Food! Food! Restaurants! Dessert! Food! Food! Drinks! Laziness!

Just listen next time you are around them, I'm sure all they do is talk about eating, drinking, relaxing, and they encourage others to do the same. They are notorious for being the pushers for bad food "OMG, this is so good taste this! Here, have a bite. I'm going to buy you a drink. Here's some more. Eat this." You know who I am talking about, because most of your friends are like this.

Their diets are terrible and the only thing they ever want to do is go out to eat and have drinks. They lack ambition to achieve any form physical levels of success for themselves. They more than likely also have either a victim mentality when it comes to fat loss or lack of belief in themselves that it is achievable. They may even be negative, excuse makers, along with binge eaters, and are definitely full-blown food addicts.

Are those the type of people you want to be around if you are trying to get shredded and successful? Is that what you want to be like in the future? Fuvk no!

So what does this mean you need to do with them? What do you need to do with the people and circles of influence that are NOT where you want to be? Eliminate. Avoid. Drastically reduce your time with these people. Yes, even if they are family.

Because if you don't, what's going to happen to your future? If you don't, are you going to be content looking like the way they look? If you don't, are you going to be happy staying where you are or worse? NO! Obvious answer, right? Yes or Yes?

Anyone that is not at the level you WANT to be at or on their way to it is holding you back. These people do not deserve to be in your presence. It may sound mean, it may sound crazy, but this is a proven FACT.

So if you are serious about getting shredded, what do you need to do? You sir, may need to make new friends. I know, I know. Your fat friends are fun, they have good time, but they are also like an anchor dropped deep in the ocean, weighing you down. They are literally stopping you from reaching your destination. They are literally dragging you down and you weren't even aware of it until now.

I would recommend having an honest talk with them and tell them that you need people around you that are going to push, encourage, support, motivate, and inspire you. If they don't honor how you feel or jump on board with you, then it's time to stop spending time with them. They obviously don't respect you, your goals or your desires to become great, so they don't belong in your life.

You don't have to avoid them forever; just keep time spent with them very rare occasions. For example, if they are super fun to party with, save those people for very special occasions that you are going to party, like your birthday, New Year's Eve, etc. Cut time spent with anyone who is average, unfit, lazy, negative, toxic, or overweight. Cut time spent with those who are not on the same path. Focus on improving your circle of influence. Improve your circles and you will improve your body and life.

I know, it is easier said than done but this is a requirement to succeed. Nothing is impossible. It's always a choice. Successful people know this, shredded people know this, and you may even know this, but you may not have thought about how it affects your physique until now. Now you know and now you are aware.

So what is the next step?

Surround yourself with success!

"Want to be amazing? Surround yourself with amazing people!"
–Joel Brown

What does this mean? It means if you want to get shredded, if you want to be wealthy, if you want to have awesome relationships, if you want a positive attitude, if you want to have an awesome life, then you have to surround yourself with people who HAVE those things. Because you become like those with whom you surround yourself.

If you want to be a millionaire? Who do you surround yourself with? Millionaires or even billionaires! Or at the very least, others who are pursuing the millionaire goals as well.

Ever notice how the wealthy only associate with other wealthy people? That's because they KNOW this principle. They know their circle of influence is the biggest determining factor to their success, so they surround themselves with other high achievers. It's not that they are stuck up; they are just focused and smart.

So if you want to get shredded, who do you surround yourself with? Shredded, ripped, fit guys! Or at the very least, someone who is serious and dedicated to creating a shredded physique just like you.

Success breeds success. Lions run with lions. Wolves run with wolves. The guy in the photo in the beginning of this chapter is my buddy Jake. Hes one of my best friends, and is my business partner. Prime example of surrounding yourself with success. Hes stays shredded year round, I stay shredded year round.

Now finding someone who is shredded may be a challenge. You may not have any friends that want to get shredded or you may not have any fit friends in your circles, so what do you do?

Fly solo until you do

If the only person you know that is working on getting shredded is you, then you ride alone. That means you spend the majority of your time with yourself, within your own thoughts, your own habits, your own behaviors, focused on YOUR training and YOUR nutrition. It is better to be alone moving forward than to be with others who pull you down.

Where is the best place to meet other fitness-minded individuals? At the gym! So make eye contact, say hello, shake some hands, or give some fist bumps daily. Create relationships with those who are dedicated, those who are shredded, and those who are consistent.

You are going to see some of the same faces day after day at the gym. Especially if you are training at the same time. So get to know these people, these are obviously dedicated, like minded, focused ambitious people. These are people you want to spend more time with. You may even pick up a new training partner.

Training partners

"A good training partner pushes you to handle more poundage and gives you incentive to grind out more reps per set. Workouts are more fun with a partner as well as more competitive. You challenge each other."
–Arnold Schwarzenegger

What is another thing that can accelerate your results and help you get shredded FASTER? What is another thing that could make you stronger quicker, and help you add more muscle to your physique faster?

Having an excellent training partner, a shredmate. Having a reliable training partner can skyrocket your success. Even Arnold Schwarzenegger trained with training partners like Franco Columbo and numerous other famous body builders of the time. So if Arnold, one of the greatest lifters of all time became successful because of using training partners, then what do you think you need to do?

You need to partner up!

Why is it more effective? Have you ever noticed that when someone is around, someone is watching, someone is spotting, you perform better? You do more reps, more weight, you keep pushing when you know you have that spotter to assist you. You really produce in training when you have someone training with you. A good training partner can increase your training efforts multiple levels and expedite your progress.

Along with pushing you harder during training, it promotes consistency, more accountability, and he can alert you to training imperfections you need to fix in your form.

With that said, I highly recommend that you partner up. But don't wait to get started. Start solo NOW and just work on improving making friends and connections and partner up over time. Finding a reliable training partner is tough, and you may have to go through a few tryouts before you find one that is adequate, so be very selective.

I also recommend a few things:

1. Surround yourself with success. You ONLY partner up with someone who is either super shredded, or working on getting super shredded. This will be someone who is dedicated, focused on the lifestyle, and is consistently reliable. Not your fat friend who is really out of shape, eats terrible, parties all the time, and is just getting started. Share this book with him, tell him to read it, then he can join you in a few months. Your training partner should be someone you want to be like, someone inspiring, someone serious, motivated, someone you know is going to push you harder. I recommend getting to know the FITTEST guy in your gym, become good friends with him and with time he may be your shredmate.

2. Be ambitious. Being that you are going to be spending a lot of time with this person, they need to be ambitious as well. They should be making around the same amount of income as you or better, or at the very least hustling to get there. No broke asses. No guys who are barely making ends meet, or are thirty-thousand-aires. Remember, we become like those we are surrounded by, so make sure he is just as ambitious as you or better, and makes six, seven, or eight figures annually.

3. Train at the right place. I also recommend training at gyms that have the more dedicated types of members. Members who actually train hard, who are motivated, who are dedicated. So don't join your local Planet Fitness or crunch gyms. These are pathetic and so are most members of those gyms. These gyms are usually full of pussies that just ACT like they are making an effort to workout. You need gyms that have BEASTS training. Gyms that have guys who are training hard, that are big, that are shredded.

You want to train is bodybuilding gyms, gyms like Gold's, or something similar, so it would be great if you have one nearby. Some 24 Hour Fitness locations (sport level and higher), are a good choice for your training. Also, training at some of the gyms that have a more affluent membership base is a great idea as well. Gyms like Equinox and most high-end sports clubs such as Life Time Athletic (of which I am a member) are great facilities to train in due to being around more affluent high achievers.

So remember, when it comes to becoming a success in getting shredded, you HAVE to surround yourself with the best. So let go of your unfit friends and find more ambitious, shredded fit friends. This is a crucial component of how fast you succeed and the height of your success.

But remember, DON'T wait until you find one. START training, eating, getting shredded now, then look for a partner over time. So get to work NOW! Now that we have discussed the importance of surrounding yourself with success, let's talk about how to socialize.

How to socialize

"Your body is a reflection of your lifestyle."
-Unknown

We are social creatures and enjoy spending time with others in fun environments. We all like to have conversations over dinner at restaurants. We all have weekend birthday parties, dinners, and events to attend. But it's only those that truly LIVE the lifestyle, those that truly do what it takes, that live shredded year-round.

You are going to have weekends full of social events all the time for the rest of your life, so I'm going to give you a few tips to help you navigate these intelligently. Understand, the rules in social situations are similar to the normal rules of nutrition. What you already know still applies. But I am going to reiterate and give you a few tips.

You should already be thinking, and living with the belief of "I don't eat that" when it comes to processed foods. You should always be making smart food choices, so eating anything with sugar or flour isn't even an option. You should still be tracking – yes, especially when you eat out at restaurants. Being shredded requires your nutrition ON POINT all the time.

That's life, so suck it up

"Consistent discipline creates consistent results."
–Daymond Sewall

Look, the reality is that you are going to be surrounded by highly addictive, fattening foods every single day for the rest of your life. Every day in your office there will be candy, donuts, birthday cake, pizza, and coffee creamers. Every time you go to a restaurant or party, there is going to be chips, pasta, bread, soda, fruit juices, alcohol, and desserts. You are going to be surrounded by this stuff every day for LIFE. So what? That's life, so suck it up!

Your bitching, whining and complaining isn't going to change anything. But what YOU can change is YOURSELF and how you behave. Starting with the "I don't eat that" mentality, followed by the EBYG strategy. For instance, let's say you have a birthday dinner for a friend to attend on Saturday. What would be the smartest way to handle this? What should you do before going so you keep your nutrition in check?

EBYG

Eat before you go. When it comes to ANY social setting, lunches, dinners, birthday parties, always, always, ALWAYS eat before you go. When I say always, I mean EVERY fuvking time. When? Always!

How often? ALWAYS!

What should you eat before you go? Good question. You should already know the answer, too. Well, what's the staple that all of your meals should consist of?

PVF

"Consistency is key."
–Unknown

Protein and veggies first. This rule ALWAYS applies, especially before attending any social gatherings, any meals out, any birthday parties, any dinners, and any event where there is alcohol involved.

Why do we EBYG? Because if you have already eaten and already put something in your stomach, you won't be hungry when you arrive. Because you won't be hungry, it is much easier to say, "No thanks, I'm full. No thanks, I already ate." It also makes it so you won't be tempted by all the junk you're going to smell and be surrounded by. So one of the biggest tricks to staying on point prior to any social event is EBYG, PVF! This one little trick makes life so much easier.

What to order

"If you are persistent you will get it. If you are consistent,
you will KEEP it."
-Unknown

Now if your calories for the day permit you can order at dinner, but what do you order? PVF! Yes, even at the restaurant order PVF. Grilled salmon, steamed asparagus. Steak and veggies. Grilled chicken and broccoli. PVF.

The reason is the food at restaurants is ALWAYS going to have MORE calories than you think it is. So even if you order grilled filet mignon with steamed veggies, that filet is probably going to have extra oils on it, traces of butter from the grill, extra ingredients, and extra calories from the way they prepare it. You have no idea what's really on it, so you really have no clue how many calories you're getting.

So always overestimate the calories when tracking restaurant food. If your MyFitnessPal says the filet is 500 calories, assume it is more like 750-1,000+ calories. Track it HIGHER than you think it is because that's more of the reality. Always play it safe, and PVF at restaurants.

Be the picky one

Because restaurants are just trying to make foods taste good so they profit more, they put terrible chemicals, ingredients in their foods to make people keep coming back. Highly addictive ingredients such as sugar and flour in the sauces, MSG, processed oils, is just naming a few. So when you are dealing with the wait staff, BE the picky one. Be the one that asks questions like, "What's in this?" Avoid sauces because of sugar and possible flour. Tell them no butter, no rub on steaks (some restaurants use flour in their rubs), and no oils -- just grilled protein and steamed veggies. Salt and pepper is fine.

Keep it simple. Keep your eating out smart and to a minimum so you can control ALL of the ingredients, weights, and macros. Obviously, the best choice is just to EBYG (eat before you go), then just go and hang out with friends and don't eat anything. But I understand we all like meals out and we all like to socialize over a meal, but just always be SMART.

If you're going somewhere you know doesn't have anything you could eat, bring your own food. EBYG, then bring another meal with you to the restaurant to eat during or after. Another simple choice is a sushi restaurant, just order sashimi. Use gluten free soy sauce(bring your own). It's very simple. Eat real food. Don't eat crap. It's simple.

"Today I will do what others won't so tomorrow I can do what others can't."
–Jerry Rice

Being shredded means living 10 levels higher than the average person and doing the opposite of what average people do. While average people are eating bread, chips, starting with drinks, consuming everything their eyes see, you DO the OPPOSITE. EBYG, drink water, socialize, make smart choices, get shredded. While average people continue to get fat, you will continue to get results.

W.O.W.

What truly separates the good physiques from the GREAT physiques? The WEEKENDS! **W.O.W.** means Work harder On Weekends.

This is where the average person ruins all of their hard work for the week. All week long they eat right, weigh portions, track food, train, then Friday rolls around and what do they do? Eat out! Drink! Mindlessly and carelessly. Then they usually do the same on Saturday and/or Sunday, only to show up at the gym on Monday FAT.

They try to fix the damage done over the weekend. They are good all week and then blow it again next weekend. It's a vicious cycle and this is one of the big reasons why you see people looking just as fat this Monday as you will next Monday. Most people make ZERO progress, and usually just continue getting fatter slowly over time with these lifestyles.

This is not you, not anymore. You are going to follow the rules and keep macros on point seven days a week. You do this by WOW. **W**orking-harder **O**n **W**eekends. Because we are social beings, there are going to be a lot of social situations you are going to have to navigate. That's life. Just know that weekends are going to require more planning, more discipline, and a bigger ball sack to say, "No thanks" quite often.

So plan ahead, follow the nutrition rules, EBYG, train before you go, and you will stay on point. This is how you get shredded and STAY shredded. Always be thinking five steps ahead.

Drinking

Would you like to know how to drink and get away with it? Would you like to know WHAT to drink so you can get away with it? Good, because I'm going to give you the tips and tricks. But first, understand drinking needs to be kept to a minimum and only on very, very rare occasions because of the effects it has on your body.

I understand, we all like to enjoy life, celebrate from time to time, have some drinks with friends. I get it. The problem is most people do it all wrong. For one, they drink too often, one to three times or more per week. Second, they drink all the wrong things. Third, they didn't prepare properly, so they set themselves up for over consuming calories, blood sugar spikes and crashes, and binge eating.

Do you know what happens to your body when you drink? Without boring you with all the science, just know this, when you ingest alcohol your body halts its fat burning until the alcohol is eliminated from your system. It sees alcohol as more of a poison, and your liver's number one priority is to eliminate it. Your shred gets slowed.

Second, it can also cause a drop in your testosterone. Not good, because we need high testosterone for fat burning, vitality, libido, and muscle development. Third, it's excess empty calories and alcohol stimulates the release of the storage hormone insulin. This sets you up for fat storing and overeating.

So knowing all of that, do you see why drinking needs to be held to very rare occasions? Good. But when it is time to drink and have some fun, there is a strategy for it. So let's teach you the smart way of drinking.

Save it for your refeed day

If you want to have drinks, schedule it on your refeed day. This is why most people do refeed days on Saturdays, because this is the day they usually are socializing, going to dinner with friends, etc. Try to always plan the days you drink as your REFEED day. You are going to be getting hundreds of extra calories from alcohol.

Do you know what that means? That means NO extra carbs for you on your refeed day because your HIGH calorie intake is coming from your alcohol. Remember, the whole point of a refeed day is to refuel, reload, and give your body a day of higher calories. The alcohol is your high calories. It's not the best quality, but it is calories.

What else should you make sure you do on this day? TRAIN! You're going to do a 1,000-calorie burn, remember?!

If we know that alcohol stimulates the release of insulin, what is a way we can help keep that in check? What should we do BEFORE we have drinks to keep our blood sugar in check?

PVF: Protein and veggies first!

This rule always applies! Before anything ever goes in your mouth, you have to PVF and this situation is no different. In order to keep blood sugar in check, keep you from over-consuming, we need to always fill your belly with PVF! Now once you have eaten PVF, what should you drink to minimize the calorie intake?

The lowest calorie options:

Straight shots (vodka, tequila, rum, etc.)
Liquor on the rocks with lime or lemon
Whiskey
Wine (in small doses)

Drinks to avoid:

Beer (because you'd have to drink a ton of them)

Mixed drinks (Long Islands, adios MF'ers, margaritas, blended, fruity drinks). These are packed with sugar worse than most sodas. So avoid any drinks, shots, that are mixed because of the sugar content. Sugar leads to cravings for more sugar.

Your alcohol choices need to be SMART, and even drinking the smart ones, you are going to get a good 400, 500, or 1,000 extra calories throughout the night, depending on your tolerance.

Have limits

With that said, keep your drinking limited. I would limit it to three to five shots, three whiskies, or three glasses of wine. Once you have hit your limit, you're done. Call Uber and go home. Along with having limits you stick to, TRACK it on your MyFitnessPal app, too.

Hydrate after each drink

Want to know how to prevent cravings? Want to know how to wake up refreshed without a hangover?

One of the reasons why you get hangovers is from dehydration. It's also one of the things that sparks cravings for carbs. So after each drink, before getting another shot, or another drink, order a bottle of water and down that between. Then right before you end the night and go to bed, guzzle another 20-40oz. You will wake up feeling fine the next day.

As always, be smart, be thinking five steps ahead, have limits, and yes, TRACK your alcohol on MyFitnessPal.

How to do holidays

When it comes to holidays, big ones like Thanksgiving, Christmas, New Year's, or any other ones that are big festivities in your life, there is a strategy to prep for them. The Holidays are typically supposed to be the time we spend with family and loved ones to show our thanks, appreciation, and celebrate. But really we all know these days have historically just turned into days of GLUTTONY. Now that you understand food and the body more, you understand why this happens. The goal for holidays is to prepare and plan ahead so that you can enjoy the holiday and stay LEAN.

Would you like to learn the tricks so you can escape being the typical American that gets fat EVERY holiday season? Would you like to learn how to navigate the holiday season and get shredded or stay shredded? Would you like to learn how you can eat pie and still stay shredded? Want to know how the fittest people stay fit year-round?

If so, I'm about to tell you the tricks so you can enjoy your holiday feasts, enjoy your family, and stay in shape. There is a step-by-step strategy you have to follow starting a week prior to prep for these holidays. You can actually even use this exact same strategy for your birthday celebration, weddings, etc.

Ready to learn it? All right, let's do this! I'm going to make this quick and list it in a few steps.

Step #1: Carb deplete.

Starting three to six days before the holiday, you are going to deplete your body of stored glycogen (carbs) by eating ONLY protein, veggies, and good fats daily. This will put you around 30g carbs a day. You eat ONLY those foods all the way up to the day of the holiday. By eating only protein, veggies, and good fats for days, it is going to deplete your muscles of the glycogen (stored carbs) so they are primed to absorb the carbs on the holiday, so you're less likely to spill over into fat. So the first step is carb depletion.

Make sure that you are still hitting the appropriate calorie intake even while doing this. When you cut carbs, your calories are going to drop, so increase your protein or fats to make up the difference. It's okay to go over on protein or fats when your carbs are lower; just stay UNDER your calorie limit.

So if your normal deficit calorie is 2,100, make sure you still get to 2,100. Just increase your fats a little bit or protein to get calories near your limit.

Foods that you CANNOT eat during this period all carbs including fruit, oats, rice, quinoa, beans or any other high carb foods.

What CAN you eat? Protein, veggies, and fats.

Protein (chicken, fish, beef, pork, shellfish, turkey, etc.)

Veggies (Eat low-carb choices such as GREENS, broccoli, asparagus, spinach, kale, lettuce, etc.)

Fats (oils, nuts, seeds, avocado, etc.)

Step #2: TRAIN! 1,000 calorie burn minimum

What happens if you don't train and you eat more calories than you burn? YOU GET FAT!!! Unacceptable! So what is the one thing you HAVE TO DO the day of your event?

Train! No excuses. IDGAF if you have to do sprints in the freezing cold or wake up at 3:00 a.m. to go get it in before everyone wakes up, DO IT! You HAVE to increase your calorie OUTPUT all week but especially on the holiday day to prevent fat gain. So if you're traveling, you had better get your ass up

EARLY that day and go TRAIN intensely before you go. You must get your calorie burn up for the day to prevent any fat gain. Plan your workout ahead of time by packing workout clothes and shoes.

Why is this so important you train on this day? Because fat gain comes from over-consuming calories. Any time you eat more calories than your body burns, it stores the excess calories as fat. So if you don't train, you're going to gain. It's very easy to gain fat if you're not burning very many calories. Get your calorie burn up as HIGH as possible to prevent any calories eaten from being stored as fat.

So what are you going to make sure you do on the day of the holiday? TRAIN!!! Burn 1,000+ calories (use a heart rate monitor to track it). Get your ass up EARLY before everyone else and go train! I don't care if you're traveling. There is a gym in every city you can train at, so pay the day fee if you're not a member. There is a high school track in every city where you can do sprints and stadiums. You can lace up your shoes, walk outside, train right out front, and do 20-50 sprints, burpees, pushups, walking lunges, etc. There is NO EXCUSE why you can't train.

Plan your workout and go DTFW so you can stay lean through the holidays.

Step #3: Protein plate FIRST!!!

All right, by this point you have been doing well, you're carb depleted, you worked out the morning of the holiday, and now it's time to enjoy the day! I actually want you to partake in some of the foods on this day. But there are rules and you need to still avoid the addictive ingredients and make your own dishes.

This rule is similar to the PVF rule, except we take it another step further. Protein plate first! Plate number one is full of PROTEIN. This means your entire first plate of food is ONLY protein. Lots of turkey, chicken, ham, eggs, or whatever else that's protein you're serving is what fills your first plate. I mean 16-24 ounces of pure protein. You do NOT touch any carbs, pie, mashed potatoes, fruit, gluten-free stuffing, or anything that has carbs until you have eaten an entire plate of your protein first.

We do this for a few reasons. First, it slows the digestion of the carbs, which will prevent your blood sugar from spiking, leading to a crash, and you eating ravenously all day (making yourself fat). Second, this is going to make you FULL all day long, which will naturally limit how much you can eat, and prevent you from overeating. You may even have what I call a "Turtle Belly." This is where you're so full your stomach sticks out and if you have abs, it will look like a turtle shell.

This rule also applies to drinking alcohol. NO DRINKS until after you have eaten your first plate of protein, for the same reason as above. No mimosas or wine until after you've eaten your first protein plate. I know in most homes, families start drinking early, so you have to wait until AFTER that protein plate. Once again, you do the OPPOSITE of what average people do.

Make sense? Good!

So what are you going to eat first? Full plate of protein!

Step #4: Make your own!

When it comes to holiday foods, most are made with the terrible ingredients that we need to avoid. This means breads, pastas, breaded foods, stuffing, pizza, pie crusts, and even the gravy all have flour or sugar or both in them. Do you remember why we avoid these?

Because number one, they are highly addictive and will lead to cravings for more refined, processed foods the rest of the day and days after. This means you will overeat and get fat. But one of the most important reasons why we also avoid them is because they are HIGHLY inflammatory and it will inflame your body from within.

This inflammation ALWAYS flares up old injuries, current muscular issues, or inflame an area that is tight and knotted already. This inflammation WILL lead to intense pain, a pulled muscle, or a torn muscle when you train next. It can limit your ability to train 100% for up to two weeks after you eat it. So avoid anything that has or could possibly have these ingredients in them. This means all the processed carbs, pie crusts, gravy, stuffing, bread, and pasta.

Want to learn how you can get to eat pie, stuffing, and other foods on these holidays? Quite simply actually, it's called make your own. Thanks to my friend Google, you can find CLEAN recipes for EVERY single dish you can imagine. The same favorite food you love, just made with healthier, smarter ingredients that won't injure you.

Want to know where to find these recipes? Want to know how to easily make pumpkin pie, apple pie, or any other dish you want? Here is the secret: you find them on Google. In the Google search bar, put in "Paleo pumpkin pie recipes" or "Paleo apple pie recipes" to find the healthy recipes for these foods. It's that easy.

The reason we search the word *Paleo* is because anything that qualifies as a Paleo food means it does not have refined flour or sugar in the ingredients. That's the standard. That's also what WE always avoid because "We don't eat that." By searching Paleo recipes, we know that we are guaranteed to get recipes that are coming from whole foods sources without all the refined sugar, refined flour, or any other processed food. There are TONS of recipe options that are super simple, using smarter ingredients, but still taste amazing.

Every year, I personally make Paleo pumpkin pies for Thanksgiving, Christmas, and they have actually become quite the hit. People actually eat more of MY pie, then they do the toxic ingredient one (that others bring).

You still must account for these calories in your MyFitnessPal. I personally make two pies, that are included in my calories for the day, just for myself. I plan these days just like a reefed: carb deplete prior, train hard the day of, just like you. Then I enjoy the holiday but still account for those pies and still make smart choices. I still keep my calories in check and always account for eating MORE than I actually do. I don't get to ever eat both of my pies because I'm too full after the protein plate, and others eat my pie, but I do make sure there is room in my calories in case I do actually eat all of both. It's better to eat less than planned than to over eat more than planned.

So that's the secret to being able to eat pie on holidays. Search "Paleo____recipe," find one that sounds the best, and give it a shot. Or you could just NOT eat at all and eat your normal meals. Or do a normal REFEED day. It's your choice.

Step #5: Be disciplined.

After you have eaten your first protein plate, you can have a little bit of the stuff you want to have! Have some Paleo pumpkin pie, mashed potatoes, Paleo stuffing, fruit salad and whatever you desire. BUT of course, there's always a BUT, BE

DISCIPLINED! Have a few bites of all the clean ingredient things you want but don't binge like a piggy.

Truly, with the first plate of protein, this is more than likely not going to be an issue, but just in case, I feel like I should mention it. Being shredded is ALL about being DISCIPLINED all the time. Don't ruin all your hard work and set yourself back weeks because you got reckless. Follow these rules and you're guaranteed to get away with it!

Truly to get shredded as fast as possible you should be weighing everything you eat, tracking, accounting for every bite. But if you follow these rules, have the initial protein-packed plate, you will naturally limit your intake. So as long as you follow all the rules, you will get through the holiday guilt-free and shredded.

Step #6: Throw it out!

This means as soon as the holiday is over, so is your eating of any holiday food. All the CARB leftovers that are there at the end of the day go straight into the TRASH. All the potatoes, pies, fruit salads, cakes, gluten-free stuffing, all the carb leftovers, go in the trash. Keep the turkey for your protein source the next few days, but all the carb foods that you might crave go in the TRASH. Toss it and you won't be tempted. Yes, I said WASTE the food.

We do this because if you don't throw it away, you're going to continue eating it and you already got your carb load. You already got to enjoy the holiday and now it's back to the grind. Trust me, it's much easier to throw these away and be disciplined with your food than it is to try and burn the fat off later. The "I'll burn it off later" mentality is why most people are always fat. This falls under the be DISCIPLINED category. Shredded people are shredded because they are highly disciplined.

Want to be shredded? Then develop high levels of discipline. So what are you going to do with all the leftovers? Good answer, throw them away! Okay, we have discussed all the different social settings that you are going to come across.

Let's Review:

1. What is the number one determining factor of the levels of success you achieve in life?
2. What should you do with your fat friends?
3. Who should you surround yourself with? Where do you find them?
4. Before going out to a dinner or social gathering, what should you do first? (Hint: EBYG)
5. Why do we do this?
6. If ordering at a restaurant, what should you order?
7. What does W.O.W. mean?
8. What should you do before drinking?
9. What's the best day to plan a day of drinking on?
10. What do you do after each drink and before bed to prevent hangover?
11. When it comes to holidays, what is the first step you should do when starting 3-6 days prior?
12. What MUST you do the day of the holiday?
13. How many calories should you burn?
14. How do you search Google for healthy recipes?
15. When the holiday is over, what do you do with all the leftover carbs?

[9]

Shredder Nutrition: Macros, Meal Plans & Tips

As promised, I'm going to make this as simple as possible because truly if you do it, this way it really is. In this chapter we are going to start bringing all the nutrition together, you're going to get your macros, get example meal plans and get more nutrition tips to help you get shredded.

Nutrition is truly very simple if you follow the rules and make all these hacks and tricks your new habits. Let's do this!

You DON'T have to eat every 2-3 hours

Wait, what??! I know, you've been told for decades that you have to eat frequently to stoke the metabolic flame and keep metabolism revving. Well, science has proven over the last few years the ONLY thing that matters is your total intake for the day and your weekly average. So it doesn't matter if you do two or six meals a day. If it is 2,100 calories, then it's 2,100 calories. The results are similar.

Although I have a plan that is five meals a day in my examples, it honestly doesn't matter if you do less meals or more, as long as your calories and macros are on point. Either three slightly bigger meals or five moderate meals will get you shredded. There is NO benefit or magic from eating six times a day like it was once thought. The key is just keeping calories on point.

Personally, I used to eat six to eight times per day years ago. It can be a pain in the ass, but it did help establish discipline, so I'm thankful for that. Now I do three to five meals a day, depending on the day, my food choices, and my phase of training. I average four meals per day and it's much easier.

Plan on eating slightly bigger meals three to five times per day or whatever fits your lifestyle the best. Four seems to be the magic number for most people, including myself. Just remember that it's all about the TOTAL calories from your macros. Keep macros on point so your calories will be on point and you get shredded.

Now that we have discussed that, let's move on to HOW to prep.

How to pack meals the easy way

See this photo? Fuvk that! This is not how we do it. You are more than welcome to, but it's not necessary.

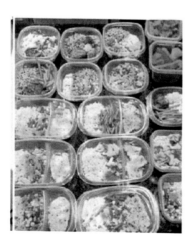

We do NOT waste our time doing this. We do NOT need to spend tons of hours completely separating each meal into its own container. Remember, it's all about the total calories and macros for the day, so here's another trick that most people aren't aware of that is MY style and is super easy: put it all into ONE container! Yep! Put all your food into ONE dish. When you eat, just eat half to one-quarter of the meal, seal it up, and eat the rest later. Wow, that's so easy! I know.

If you are going to be away from home for work, you may need one to three meals to take with you. Pack it all in ONE dish and you're set!

For example:

Old School Meal Prep (we don't do this)

You have tons of containers and let's say you need to take three meals to work.

- Container #1
  6 oz. chicken, 200 g veggies, 100 g brown rice

- Container #2
  6 oz. chicken, 200 g veggies, 100 g brown rice

- Container #3
  6 oz. chicken, 200 g veggies, 1 oz. nuts

This is 3 meals in 3 separate containers. That is fine because it is great for establishing self-discipline, but is unnecessary to get shredded.

Shredder Style Meal Prep

Just like how I give you all the tricks and hacks to make getting shredded simplified, here is another one. This is the same calories and same macros, just in one container.

In one large container:
18 oz. chicken, 600 g veggies, 200 g brown rice, 1 oz. nuts

When it's time to eat, eat 1/3-1/2 of it. Done! So easy, right? But remember, what's the number one rule when it comes to eating?

#1 Rule: PVF

The rule ALWAYS applies: protein and veggies first. Always eat your protein and veggies FIRST, because they are the most important and they will slow the digestion of any carbs you eat. This will stimulate the release of the proper hormones at the proper levels, give you very stable blood sugar levels, give you great energy, make you fuller longer, and keep you on point. Keeping your hormones and blood sugar in check are key to your success.

So that's the trick to easily packing your food. Get a good size container, pack up all your food in ONE container. I like to put my protein on one side of the container, then the veggies and carbs on the other.

Simple, right? Good.

How to weigh portions

"The price of being shredded is called DISCIPLINE."
–Daymond Sewall

When it comes to being accurate so your calories and macros are on point, I recommend always WEIGHING your portions in ounces or grams. Proteins is in ounces, then always do your fats and carbs in grams.

The reason is because this is much more accurate than doing 1 Tbsp., 1 cup, or ½ cup, versions. That one cup of rice could be a HEAPING cup, which is more likely to be the case, which means you're getting 10-20% more calories, fats, or carbs than you think. Yeah you, I'm talking to you. I know everyone always wants to eat MORE than they should and lives in denial about how much they eat. So to be super accurate and WEIGH your portions.

Proteins weighed in ounces or grams, if you prefer. Carbs and fats definitely are weighed in grams.

Proteins

When it comes to weighing your portions, technically the nutritional info on the packaging and the MyFitnessPal app typically refers to the food weighed RAW. So when you see a nutritional value of say chicken thighs at 140 calories for 4 ounces, this is referring to it in raw form. When you cook the chicken, it could lose up to 50% of its weight.

So to be safe and always accurate, weigh all your protein portions RAW. If you are going to eat 16 ounces of chicken for a couple of your meals, weigh it out BEFORE cooking. You want accuracy at all times. Even though it is protein, if you eat

16 ounces cooked when really it was 32 ounces because it lost 50% of its weight during cooking, you just ate 1,120 calories of chicken instead of the 560 calories you tracked. By doing that, you could get fat or not lose very much fat. Weigh it raw to be accurate.

This is especially crucial when eating protein sources that are higher in fat, like grass-fed ground beef, ground turkey, chicken thighs, and salmon, because these sometimes lose a lot of weight after cooking. I know, it may sound like its tedious, but that's the price of SUCCESS. You've got to DTFW!

But I do actually have some hacks for you. Want to know an easy hack for the ground meats? Want to know one of my secrets? Buy the prepackaged 16 ounce versions, some of these come in precut 4 ounce patties.

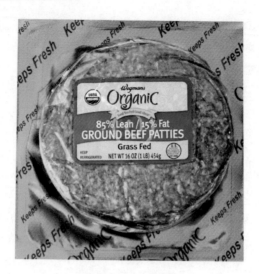

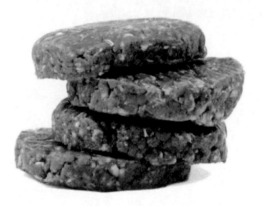

This makes it super easy to track and prep. Each patty is 4 ounces worth of protein. This is the simple way of eating ground meats. You can do the same with turkey, chicken, lamb, and any other ground meats there are. Just look around for them and you'll find them.

Cooking in bulk hack

When cooking up things like chicken, steak, or pork, the simple hack to cook in bulk is to cook up 5-10 pounds, then just split it up into 5-10 equal parts. Let's say you weighed five pounds of protein and cooked it up, so it's obviously going to weigh less than five pounds after. Just split the cooked meat into five equal parts and put them into separate containers or freezer bags in fridge. If you get 15 ounces in one container one day and 17 ounces in the next, it's not going to make that big of a difference. Your deficit average for the week will be the same.

By doing it this way, you already know you have about a pound in each one, then prepping each night for the next day is easier, you just toss in the other stuff you need with it. So that's the simple hack for cooking up chicken, pork, and steak. As you start gaining experience, you will start to create your own little systems of doing things. I'm just giving you a few ideas, but feel free to modify to fit your life. Just make sure you are being accurate.

Bulk patties

You can also cook up lots of the precut patties in bulk. These make for quick and easy prep as well. You know each one is going to be 4 ounces, so the measuring has been done. All you have to do is track it.

Eggs hack

This is one of the easiest hacks to prep and track because they are already premeasured for you by the shell. They are the same calories and macros for each. What I recommend is boiling up two to three dozen eggs, peeling them, then placing them in a storage container in fridge. This is another hack to make meal prep a cinch.

Personally, I like to have a few protein sources made at all times so I have options. I usually always have eggs peeled in bulk in fridge. I usually have a supply of beef patties made. Being an entrepreneur, doing most of my work from my home office, I actually get to eat most of my meals out of my home. So even though I have stuff prepped, I also get to cook most of my meals fresh throughout the day. You may not have that luxury, so cook up a few in bulk.

Carbs

When it comes to carbs, these get weighed in grams. These are very easy to weigh when you're eating fruit or potatoes of any kind, because fruit is weighed raw and potatoes keep about the same weight after cooking. But when you are weighing things that require water and swell once cooked like rice or quinoa, these are measured and tracked in their cooked form.

Later on in this chapter, I have example meal plans, when you see the measurements on the nutrition examples like "100 g brown rice," this refers to the cooked version. But I will specify on those as well, so just pay attention.

Oats are one of the only exceptions. I personally am not a fan of oats but if you are, these portions are weighed dry before cooking. Chances are you won't want oats now that you can't add sweeteners to them anyway.

Fats

When dealing with fat sources, these are weighed on the scale in grams as well. Fats are vital to your shreds but they are also very calorie dense. It is very, very easy to over-consume eating fats. So when dealing with these, always weigh them in grams.

Keep in mind that 28 grams = 1 ounce. For most of your fat sources like oils, nuts, and butter, they will be in 7 gram to 28 gram servings. Accuracy is key to creating a deficit to melt fat off your body. Be obsessive. As you start getting some experience and habits develop, it gets easier.

How to track

When tracking food, always make sure you track the correct BRAND. Chicken from one farm will have completely different nutritional info than chicken from another farm. Make sure you do your homework and track the correct one.

For instance, if you're eating Organic Tyson Chicken Thigh, in the search category of the MFfitnessPal app, search "Organic Tyson Chicken Thigh," not just "chicken thigh." You will see the nutritional info varies greatly between some brands. Track accurately.

One brand could be 120 calories for 4 ounces, while another could be 210 calories for 4 ounces. Add this up over the period of a day and you could easily be eating 300,400, or over 500 extra calories per day if you're logging the wrong brand. So pay attention and do your homework. Look on their websites and create your OWN food in the app if you have to.

Prep each night

Prep food each night for the next day. Every night before you go to bed, pack up your food for the next day at work, weigh it out, track it on MyFitnessPal, and put it in a container so it's ready to grab and go in the morning. You can also add your breakfast to this container, so you can just wake up, eat, and go.

Remember, you can store it all in one container; you don't have to have five separate containers. Just make sure you weigh it all out, track it, and eat your protein and veggies first. First, put in veggies and carbs, weigh them out, then hit the "clear" or "Tare" button to zero out the food scale, and then put in your protein. This puts your protein on top because it's priority.

For example, let's say you're packing 16 oz. chicken thighs, 300 g broccoli, and 500 g watermelon. Place the watermelon in the dish and weigh out 500 g. Then hit the Tare button. This will zero out the food scale with your plate with the food in it, then add your 300 g of broccoli. Hit the Tare button to zero it out again. Then add in your chicken. Done! It's super easy!

Or if you already had the chicken in a container in a one-pound portion, just follow the first two steps for the watermelon and broccoli. Alternately, you could just keep them in a separate container and you just have two large containers. It's your choice. I'm giving you the easy hacks, but you must make it work for your lifestyle.

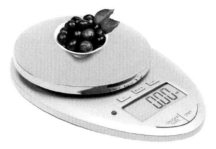

How to use MyFitnessPal

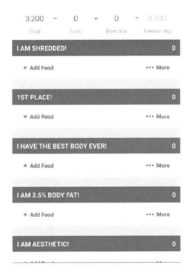

These are the names of my five meals. You don't have to track each meal separately, so you can actually just add it all under ONE meal. I usually just put all of my meals under the "I am Shredded" meal tab. The total numbers, macros, and calories will still be the same; it just makes it quicker to do it under one meal.

When adding foods, a lot of them that come in packages like the beef patties, turkey patties, and oats, you can scan a barcode and it will pull up the info for you. If you look on the right-hand side of this picture, you'll see the barcode. Just click that and scan the barcode, then add the food. This app also keeps your most recent foods on a list for easy updating on a daily basis.

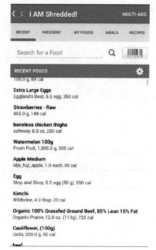

When searching for foods that do not have a barcode, like some protein sources, fruit, and veggies, in the top left you can "Search For Food." Like I said, When you "search for food," be very specific with the type of food, the brand, and the measurement. The results with the green check mark mean they are verified and accurate.

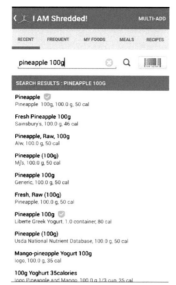

Look for the green checks, but if there's not any, find the one that is YOUR personal brand that is accurate. You can create your own food in the app if you have to. When you track your food like right here where I tracked my breakfast, make sure you are very accurate with your weights so your macros are on point.

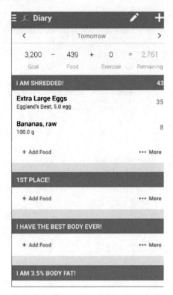

How to see macros

Once you have entered your foods with the right measurements, you can take a peek at your macros by going to the "Nutrition" tab on the home screen of MyFitnessPal. There are a few different pages now and the app is constantly being improved. But this screen below is a pie chart showing your percentage of each macro and the grams eaten so far. As you can see with the 5 eggs and 100 g banana I have tracked, it keeps track of your macros and calories. So far I have eaten 23 g carbs, 23 g fats, and 36 g protein.

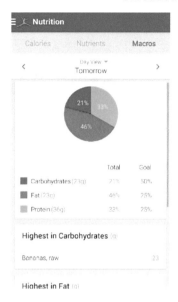

There is another screen that shows your macros and micros, your goal amounts, and how much you have remaining. This is the page you want to be paying the most attention to. Your goal is to get as close to your goal macros as possible but staying slightly UNDER your calories.

It's okay if you're off by a couple grams here and there; just make sure you are prioritizing your protein and fats. NEVER go over your carbs or your calories. It's okay to be a little higher in fats and protein if your carbs are lower. Especially in Phases Two and Three of the eating plan. Increase your fats to increase your calories. Just always make sure you stay just a smidge UNDER your recommended deficit calories.

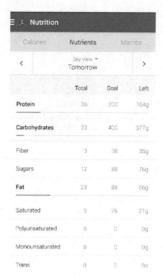

Want to know what one of the best habits to get into is?

The best time to track

Want to know the best time to track for optimal accuracy? Want to know how to prevent making mistakes and over eating? It's simple: develop the habit of tracking BEFORE you eat. Get in the habit of weighing portions and tracking your food BEFORE you eat it. This will keep you from making a mistake and overeating by accident. Make it a habit to track it and check your numbers BEFORE you eat.

Master these two skills of weighing and tracking and you will master your results. Remember, your results are the sum total of HOW YOU EAT. Master this and YOU'VE GOT THIS!

Flavoring

When it comes to eating healthy, it doesn't have to be boring. You can actually create some awesome dishes using all-natural ingredients. The key is to just experiment. Mix together different onions, peppers, herbs, spices, and play with it. Sometimes it comes out the bomb and other times it sucks. This is how you learn what you like and don't like.

Typical seasonings you will find at stores have forms of sugar, processed oils, and even flour in the ingredients. Check the ingredients and throw away any that have oils, sugar, or anything you don't know what it is. It should only have herbs, spices, peppers, and salt in ingredients.

The best and cleanest seasonings on the market I have found to date are Flavorgod seasonings. You can get these online at www.Flavorgod.com I have a cabinet full of them.

Here are the must-haves in your kitchen for flavor:

- Frank's Original hot sauces, organic salsa, mustard (no sugar), Chalula, Tapatio, and Rau's Marinara.
- Himalayan salt, pepper, cayenne, turmeric, cumin, and any other herb or spice you like.

But because I'm expediting your learning curve, here are some combination hacks:

- On boiled eggs: Mustard with Frank's is bomb! Salsa or marinara also work.
- On chicken: Turmeric chicken is my favorite. Cook on the stove covered and put tons of turmeric on both sides of the chicken, then salt.
- On beef: All the red sauces. Flavorgods. Always salt.
- On turkey: Turmeric or Flavorgods. Always salt.

Like I said, play with it, experiment. What I like versus what you may like may differ. If it's good, eat it. If it sucks, eat it but don't make it again. Try something else next time.

Make sure that you TRACK the marinara and oils or butters you cook with. These calories DO count. Everything adds up!

Expect and seek the naysayers

When you begin this journey and start training hard, consistently, and start making smart nutritional choices, you are going to get pushback. The people around you are going to start throwing rocks at you via words. Expect it.

How to deal with the naysayers

Look, in order to get this physique, you are going to have to become literally OBSESSED about getting it. You're going to have to obsess over your food, obsess over your choices, the portions, the types of foods and you're going to have to say, "No thank you" a lot to food, dinners, and drinks. You're going to have to be obsessed about getting your training in DAILY. Obsessed about improving yourself, lifting better, stricter, more weight, pushing your limits, and continually improving. Being obsessed is not a bad thing; it's a REQUIREMENT to succeed.

Know that when you start this journey, your partner/spouse/friends/family/coworkers are going to give you shit. They are going to make fun, throw stones, and talk crap, to try and bring you down – down to their level. The reason they do this is because your actions, disciplines, choices, and behaviors are a mirror reflection of their flaws and weaknesses. It's a reflection of their failures, their lack of belief in themselves, their lack of discipline, their fat, their insecurities.

They don't like feeling like they are flawed and failing alone, and they fear that you will succeed and leave them behind, so they run their mouths. They are trying to talk you down to bring you back to their level. Know that this IS GOING to happen. Expect it. Expect to travel this road alone at first. Don't let their words pull you down or slow you down. Just put your eyes straight and focus on the process!

Getting this physique literally means doing the OPPOSITE of what average people do. If you do average people things, you look like average people. Average people are FAT and 95% of Americans are fat/overweight/obese. Who the fuvk wants to be average?!

> ### *"Being average is the worst thing you can be."*
> ### *- Arnold Schwarzenegger*

So when average people are eating lunch, eating out, eating candy at their desk, eating cake or bagels in the break room, having drinks multiple times per week, DON'T be average. Just look at their behaviors and their bodies. Do you want to look like that? I think not. So don't do what they do; do the opposite.

So how do you deal with them? Train daily. Pack your meals. Hit your macros. Stay on point every day, seven days a week. Remember, you become like those you surround yourself with, so if they aren't helping you move forward, cut them from your life. Surround yourself with winners.

It will swing back

In a few months when they see how awesome you're looking, they start seeing how confident you are with a big smile on your face because of your inner pride, your increased self-esteem and happiness, they are going to go from talking crap to asking you HOW you did it. It will swing back. All the shit talkers will switch from throwing stones and trying to sabotage you to swinging back around and start asking you questions on HOW TO do it. This is GUARANTEED!

This is how it works for everyone. They get haters and naysayers in the first few months, but as long as you keep moving forward, keep making progress, keep getting those shreds, and these same naysayers will become ADMIRERS. Admirers that start asking for tips, tricks, and if they can work out with you. Admirers that get inspired FROM YOU. One of the most incredible things about getting shredded is how inspiring you become to others.

You taking care of yourself makes others want to raise their standards to another level. It makes others feel like it's possible and believe in themselves more. I promise your haters and naysayers will come back around to becoming inspired admirers. Your success will instill belief into them that THEY too can achieve it.

So if you're getting comments like, "You're obsessed. You're crazy. Live a little. (This one always comes from fatties). You can skip this workout. Stop being so picky. Just one bite. You're a maniac." The list goes on. GOOD! This means you are on the right track. If you aren't getting comments like this or negative ones from people trying to talk you down, then you're NOT DOING ENOUGH.

If you're not getting rocks thrown from average people, then that means your actions are AVERAGE. You're doing the same things the average people are doing. Because if you are rising above mediocrity, you will hear it from all the peasants. Your job is to be so fuvking obsessed that you DO get these comments. If you're not, WORK HARDER and be more disciplined! Be the mirror that reflects their flaws, be the disciplined one that does the opposite, and inspire them over time to BE BETTER.

Okay, we have covered the basics, now let's get into the actual numbers and nutrition plans!

Calorie and macro cheat sheet

"The results you get from this program will be the sum total of all of your food choices."
-Tom Venuto

Your results with this program will be the sum total of all of your food choices. Your current body is the result of your past food choices. Your current health is the sum result of all of your food choices. Everything that you eat ADDS up. Everything that you consume adds to the total calorie intake for the day, and everything you eat is either benefitting you or damaging you. Getting shredded requires you spend most days deficiting so you have to always be mindful and know exactly what you're getting from your food.

I'm a huge fan of carb cycling. Simply put, this is a type of dieting that has periods of lower or moderate carb days, followed by a higher calorie carb refeed day. This is split up into three phases of carb cycling, with fat burning days (creating a deficit) and refeed days. As the phases progress, your carbs are lower on deficit days, but a little higher on refeed days. Remember that if you are leaner, you're doing six days of low carbs, with the seventh day higher (refeed). If you're heavier, do 13 days low, and the fourteenth day is higher carbs (refeed).

To simplify this, it is split up by height. Your height is a general determining factor of the average guy's build and gives a good estimate of your possible BMR. These numbers represent my recommendations for you based on your height. I don't factor into account age or weight because this is all about simplicity. Regardless of your body type, this WILL get you shredded. So do as directed and you will look and feel better than you ever expected. These calories and macros are going to get you SHHHHREEEDDDDED!

Look for your recommended calories for your height, then look at the MyFitnessPal percentage recommendations so you can customize it in your app.

To customize your MyFitnessPal:

Step 1: Go to home screen by hitting the lines in top left corner for most phones.

Step 2: Go to the "Goals" tab

Step 3: Go to the "Calorie and Macronutrient Goal" section and input the percentages I've given you here.

Now that Under Armour owns it, they have just made a feature where you can set daily goals too if you sign up for the upgraded version. You can set your refeed day numbers, too. It's pretty cool.

Now lets move on to the actual nutrition, calorie and macro recommendations that are going to get you shredded!

Deficit Calories and Macros

Phase #1 (Day 1-30)
Moderate carb deficit calories and macros
Eat this amount of calories for 6-13 days straight, then refeed on the 7th or 14th day

MyFitnessPal Percentages: 20% carbs, 40% protein, 40% fats

Height	Daily Calories	Protein	Carbs	Fats
5'4" and under	1,900	190 g	95 g	85 g
5'5" - 5'6"	2,100	210 g	105 g	94 g
5'7" - 5'9"	2,200	220 g	110 g	98 g
5'10" - 5'11"	2,300	230 g	115 g	102g
6'0" - 6'2"	2,400	240 g	120 g	107 g
6'3" - 6'5"	2,600	260 g	130 g	116 g
6'5" or over	2,800	280 g	140 g	125 g

It is best to center your meals that have slightly higher carbs right around your workouts, meaning that you should have 30-40 grams of carbs before and after training. This gives you energy for training and gives you carbs to help with post-workout recovery. The rest of your meals should just contain protein, veggies, fats.

Below I have an example meal plan for the average guy eating 2,100 calories per day. Now, I'm not going to put meal plans for each guy or calorie intake, because the reality is that it wouldn't be accurate anyway. Remember, the brands have different macros and calories. Plus, I have found over my years in training that even though I do write all my clients' personalized meal plans, they ALWAYS end up making up their own. They just follow the simple eating rules and hit their macros.

Below, I'm just giving you an example of what your day would look like as a guide to give you a visual representation of how to eat to get shredded. Remember, it doesn't have to be five meals a day and you can pack it all in one container. I'm just doing this for the sake of simplicity.

"Nutrition is EVERYTHING."
-Daymond Sewall

A typical day of eating five meals that total 2,100 calories for someone who works out in the morning would look like this:

Meal #1: 5 whole eggs, veggies, pre-workout carbs 400 g strawberries
Meal #2: 6 oz. chicken, Veggies, post-workout carbs 200 g bananas
Meal #3: 6 oz. chicken, veggies, 1 oz. nuts
Meal #4: 6 oz. ground beef, veggies, 1 Tbsp. grass-fed butter
Meal #5: 6 oz. ground beef, veggies, 1 Tbsp. grass-fed butter

Remember, it doesn't have to be five meals. It can be three or four if that's what fits your lifestyle best. Just eat bigger meals, spaced four to five hours apart and stay under your calorie limits. It's all about the total numbers for the day. So if you want to do three meals, then do that. If you want to do four meals, then do four meals. Find what works for you and stick to it. For me, it's four meals per day. You stay in a deficit for 6-13 days, then do a reefed day.

Don't be surprised if you are full when you first start doing this, because it is normal. Healthy, high-quality food is filling. It is slower to digest, triggers the release of the right hormones, and keeps you fuller. You will adapt over time and might start feeling hungry sometimes when you're burning fat, especially as you get leaner.

Refeed Days for Phase #1 (Days 1-30)

Refeeds are to be done every seventh or fourteenth day. Lean guys take the seventh day; heavy guys every fourteenth day.

MyFitnessPal percentages: 45% carbs, 30% protein, 25% fats.

Note: Always eat protein first every meal. Regardless of the carb and fat macros, stay UNDER your calorie limit.

Height	Daily Calories	Protein	Carbs	Fats
5'4" and under	2,500	188 g	282 g	69 g
5'5" - 5'6"	2,600	195 g	293 g	72 g
5'7" - 5'9"	2,900	218 g	327 g	80 g
5'10" - 5'11"	3,000	225 g	338 g	83 g
6'0" - 6'2"	3,200	240 g	361 g	89 g
6'3" - 6'5"	3,500	263 g	394 g	97 g
6'5" and over	3,700	277 g	417 g	102 g

Typically on a refeed day, the two primary macros to focus on are protein and carbs. This day, you reduce your fats a bit. For the avg guy, at 2100 days deficit, his refeed day would be around 2900. Remember that on refeed days, you MUST burn 1,000+ calories in training. His refeed looks like this below.

Refeed 2900 Calories

Meal #1: 5 whole eggs, veggies, 400 g strawberries
Meal #2: 6 oz. chicken, veggies, 225 g bananas
Meal #3: 6 oz. chicken, veggies, 200 g quinoa
Meal #4: 6 oz. ground beef, veggies, 200 g quinoa
Meal #5: 6 oz. ground beef, veggies, 2 apples.

Phase #2 (Days 29-56)
Low/moderate Carb

Eat this amount of calories for 6-13 days straight, then refeed on Day 7 or 14. All we are doing is reducing the carbs a bit, then increasing fats to make up the difference.

MyFitnessPal Percentages: 15% carbs, 40% protein, 45% fats

Height	Daily Calories	Protein	Carbs	Fats
5'4" and under	1,900	190 g	71 g	95 g
5'5" - 5'6"	2,100	210 g	79 g	105 g
5'7" - 5'9"	2,200	220 g	82 g	110 g
5'10" - 5'11"	2,300	230 g	86 g	115 g
6'0" - 6'2"	2,400	240 g	90 g	120 g
6'3" - 6'5"	2,600	260 g	97 g	130 g
6'5" and over	2,800	280 g	105 g	140 g

A typical day of eating five meals per day or 2,100 calories for someone who works out in the morning would look like this:

Meal #1: 5 whole eggs, veggies, pre-workout carbs
300 g strawberries
Meal #2: 6 oz. chicken, veggies, post-workout carbs
150 g bananas
Meal #3: 6 oz. chicken, veggies, 2 oz. nuts
Meal #4: 6 oz. ground beef, veggies, 1 Tbsp. grass-fed butter
Meal #5: 6 oz. ground beef, veggies, 1 Tbsp. grass-fed butter

REFEEDS for Phase #2 (Day 29-56)

Refeeds to be done every seventh or fourteenth day. Lean guys on Day 7, heavy guys on Day 14.

Note: Always eat protein first every meal. Regardless of the carb and fat macros, stay UNDER your calorie limit.

MyFitnessPal percentages: 45% carbs, 30% protein, 25% fats.

Height	Daily Calories	Protein	Carbs	Fats
5'4" and under	2,500	188 g	282 g	69 g
5'5"- 5'6"	2,600	195 g	293 g	72 g
5'7"- 5'9"	2,900	218 g	327 g	80 g
5'10"- 5'11"	3,000	225 g	338 g	83 g
6'0"-6'2"	3,200	240 g	361 g	89 g
6'3"-6'5"	3,500	263 g	394 g	97 g
6'5" and over	3,700	277 g	417 g	102g

A typical reefed day that is five meals equivalent to 2,900 calories per day would look like this:

Meal #1: 5 whole eggs, veggies, 400 g strawberries
Meal #2: 6 oz. chicken, veggies, 225 g bananas
Meal #3: 6 oz. chicken, veggies, 225 g quinoa
Meal #4: 6 oz. ground beef, veggies, 225 g quinoa
Meal #5: 6 oz. ground beef, veggies, 2 apples

Phase #3 Low Carb (day 57-90+)

Stay on for 6 days, refeed on Day 7.
The macros are 5% carbs, 45% protein, 50% fats (leafy green veggies only as carbs).

Height	Daily Calories	Protein	Carbs	Fats
5'4" and under	1,900	213 g	24 g	106 g
5'5" - 5'6"	2,100	236 g	26 g	117 g
5'7" - 5'9"	2,200	247 g	28 g	122 g
5'10" - 5'11"	2,300	258 g	29 g	128 g
6'0" - 6'2"	2,400	269 g	30 g	133 g
6'3" - 6'5"	2,600	292 g	33 g	145 g
6'5" and over	2,800	314 g	35 g	156 g

A typical day of eating five meals per day or 2,100 calories for someone who works out in the morning would look like this:

Meal #1: 5 whole eggs, veggies, 15 fish oil pills
Meal #2: 6 oz. chicken, veggies, 1 Tbsp. olive oil
Meal #3: 6 oz. chicken, veggies, 2 oz. nuts
Meal #4: 6 oz. ground beef 85/15, veggies,
1 Tbsp. grass-fed butter
Meal #5: 6 oz. ground beef 85/15, veggies,
1 Tbsp. grass-fed butter

Refeed Day for Phase #3 (Days 57-90+)

MyFitnessPal percentages: 50% carbs, 30% protein,
20% fats

Note: Always eat protein first at every meal. Regardless of the carb and fat macros, stay UNDER your calorie limit.

Height	Daily Calories	Protein	Carbs	Fats
5'4" and under	2,500	188 g	313 g	55 g
5'5" - 5'6"	2,600	195 g	325 g	57 g
5'7" - 5'9"	2,900	218 g	363 g	64 g
5'10" - 5'11"	3,000	226 g	375 g	66 g
6'0" - 6'2"	3,200	241 g	400 g	71 g
6'3" - 6'5"	3,500	263 g	438 g	77 g
6'5" and over	3,700	278 g	463 g	82 g

A typical refeed day Phase #3 consists of five meals or 2,900 calories would look like this:

Meal #1: 5 whole eggs, veggies, 500 g strawberries
Meal #2: 6 oz. chicken, veggies, 250 g bananas
Meal #3: 6 oz. chicken, veggies, 250 g quinoa
Meal #4: 6 oz. ground beef, veggies, 250 g quinoa
Meal #5: 6 oz. ground beef, veggies, 2 apples

These phases of calories and macros WILL GET YOU SHREDDED like a high-quality chisel! You just have to be consistent.

Notice the one thing that is common every single meal? protein and veggies. These are the staples at EVERY meal. Get creative with how you cook and flavor food. Try different combinations of veggies, herbs, and spices.

Getting shredded is purely all about consistency and consistently creating a caloric deficit by hitting your macros. Obsessively weigh foods, track your intake, and be conscious of every single bite you put in your mouth. Everything counts! Nutrition is EVERYTHING! This is why we are spending so much time educating you and teaching you the tricks nutritionally.

So those are the 3 phases of nutrition. The key points to remember is that its ALL about your calories and macros. Always stay under your calorie limits, always prioritize your protein and fats. Always keep your nutrition on point. Do that and you are guaranteed to get shredded!

"Being shredded means being on point seven days a week."
–Daymond Sewall

Let's Review:

1. True or false? You have to eat every two to three hours.
2. What is the magic number of meals per day for most people?
3. How do we pack meals the easy way?
4. Is protein weighed in grams or ounces?
5. Are carbs and fats weighed in grams or ounces?
6. Is protein weighed raw or cooked?
7. What is the hack for ground meats?
8. What is the hack for eggs?
9. Are brown rice and quinoa weighed cooked or raw?
10. How many grams equal one ounce?
11. What is the most important thing you must do when tracking food on MyFitnessPal?
12. When do you pack your food?
13. When is the best time to track your food on MyFitnessPal?
14. What do typical seasonings have in ingredients that you need to avoid?
15. What are five things you should have in your kitchen to add flavor to your food?
16. What should you expect from average people? If it's not happening, what does it tell you that you need to do?
17. Finish this quote: "Being average is the……"
18. In a few months, what will happen to the people who were the naysayers?
19. What is carb cycling?

20. What are your personal macros for deficit days and refeed days?

21. Finish this quote: "Being shredded means being......"

[10]

How to Train to Get Shredded

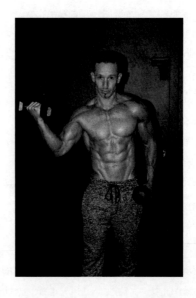

In this chapter, we are going to discuss HOW to train. Some of the things you are going to hear are going to be the opposite of what you think or have heard and it's going to cut through all the misinformation and just give you the facts on what you need to know. I PERSONALLY use these methods and use them to get my clients shredded. They fuvking work! So forget what you know, forget what you have heard, and just open your mind and absorb this like a sponge. I am about to make your training INTENSE but fun and extremely effective. All of this is scientifically proven and proven through experience.

"Do as directed and you will look and feel better than you ever expected."
–Daymond Sewall

Don't Do Cardio!

I know what you're thinking. "Wait, What?! I thought we were trying to get shredded? Don't we need to do cardio to burn fat?" NO!

For some reason, every time someone thinks about losing weight and burning fat, they immediately think about doing lots of cardio. They think they need to spend 60 minutes a day running on a frickin' treadmill or spend 45 minutes on a damn stepmill twice a day, wasting time like a hamster on a wheel, or running marathons to burn fat. This type of cardio is called LISS: Low Intensity Steady State cardio.

Fat burning zone myth

The old "Fat burning zone" BS, I'm sure you have heard it and use it. If you haven't, let me give you a quick rundown. During training, your body draws energy from primarily two places: fat or glycogen stores. Glycogen is just stored carbs in your muscles and liver.

The fat burning zone was conceived because at lower intensities, more fat is burned relative to glycogen. For example, when you are at around 50% of your max heart rate, your body burns a ratio of 60% fat to 40% glycogen. If you train at 75% of your max heart rate, the ratio is about 35% fat, 65% glycogen, so the ratio is lower. Sounds like a win, huh? You get to walk on a treadmill and burn more fat.

Not so fast. If it was that easy, there would be a lot more ripped guys walking around. You see, when you train at a low intensity, you are BARELY burning any calories; when you train hard, you burn A LOT of calories.

Now with what you know so far about burning fat, what is the key to making it happen? What state do you need to be in to force your body to burn fat? A DEFICIT. If your pansy ass is walking on a treadmill for 30 minutes, do you honestly think you are going to burn very many calories? How big of a deficit do you think you are going to create? Not much.

You see, the most important element isn't where your calories come from during training. What's important is the TOTAL burn for the day. The bigger the deficit, the MORE fat your body is going to burn off throughout the day.

For instance, take two guys named Badass Bob and Princess Pete. Bob does 30 minutes of 50-yard sprints. Bob is going to burn 400-700 calories, depending on his size and effort. Princess walks on a treadmill for 30 minutes. Princess is going to burn 200 calories.

Who do you think is going to get shredded faster? It's kind of obvious now, huh? This is why the fat burning zone is bullshit. I could write a book on this topic alone but to spare your time, just know that it's all about the TOTAL burn for the day. We want to have HIGH calorie outputs each day to create an awesome deficit to burn fat.

Let's get back to why else LISS isn't a good choice.

So let me ask you this: Is being skinny fat or having arms and legs like a 14 year-old girl your goal? Is being ravenously hungry from the increased hunger your goal? Is having low testosterone levels your goal? Is slowing your metabolism and ruining your BMR your goal? Is it your goal to accelerate aging?

No, right?

Then STOP doing Low Intensity Steady State cardio! Because that is what steady state cardio and endurance style cardio is going to do to you. It's going to make you hungrier, set you up for fat storing, become a more efficient calorie burner (burn less calories), it's going to stimulate muscle wasting, giving you skinny arms and legs, it's going to accelerate aging making you look older, and due to the muscle loss and adaptation, it will reduce your BMR and make your metabolism slower.

That's the OPPOSITE of what we want, right? Know this: you can get ripped doing literally ZERO traditional cardio. Yes, I said ZERO cardio. How is that? If your diet is on point like I have been teaching you in this book, all you have to do is intense weight training the way I am going to teach you, and you will melt fat, get shredded, and look like a GOD. We don't need, nor do we do steady state, low intensity, or endurance forms of cardio.

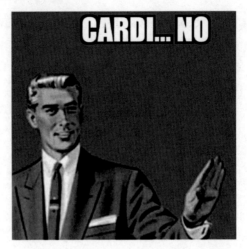

Do you ever see any other lean animals in the wild running for hours and hours? No, we are the only animal that does this terrible form of activity. Why spend a cheesy, time-wasting workout to get hardly any calorie burn, that could waste your hard earned muscle, and piss away your valuable TIME?! Wouldn't you prefer workouts that promote muscle maintenance and get you shredded?

We want workouts that create fat burning, muscle developing hormones like testosterone and growth hormone, right? We want workouts that are going to spike metabolism and continue to keep burning more fat even after we are done right? (This is the afterburn effect.) We want workouts that are going to save us TIME spent training so we can continue to grow our businesses and live our lives, right or right?

What would you say if I told you that the science and research has proven time and time again that High Intensity Interval Training is the MOST effective form of cardio to melt fat? This is why if we are going to do any form of cardio, we do ONLY HIIT forms of cardio! The ONLY forms of cardio you should ever do, is High Intensity Interval Training. HIIT does exactly all of the things our bodies are designed to do, short bursts of intense work followed by a recovery. We don't even call HIIT cardio, we call it "Conditioning"

An easy example of conditioning is sprints. Like to run? Cool. Lace up, go outside, warm up, pick a point 50 yards away, sprint down, and jog or walk back. Repeat until you've done it 20-50 times. This will take you merely 10-30 minutes and will have you looking for a bush to puke in. This is how you create an afterburn effect for up to 24+ hours. This is how you melt fat, train quickly to promote testosterone and growth hormone, how you do cardio to KEEP and even increase your muscle, and how you save TIME training. This is how you develop a SHREDDED physique. Time is money and training at a high intensity is money for your results.

Look at the best physiques of top-level athletes, what do you think they do daily? How do you think these athletes train? They sprint and LIFT. Some of the BEST physiques in the world come from top level sprinters.

Which body is best for health and performance?

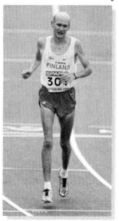 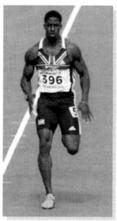

Just look at this example of a marathon runner and sprinter. The marathon runner has tiny, emaciated chest, back, legs, and is aging rapidly, looking terribly old. The sprinter looks young, vibrant, very muscular, and well developed, and he is RIPPED. Which physique would you rather have? The sprinter, or the sprinter? I thought so. NO frickin' endurance training or Low Intensity Steady State cardio.

Also keep in mind, you will hear a lot of physique athletes talk about doing steady state cardio on social media and other sites, but KNOW that the majority of these people are NOT natural. They take performance enhancing drugs, which is helps them grow and retain muscle when they do long bouts of cardio. It's the drugs developing that physique, not them. A natural guy doing the same thing is likely to end up losing a lot of muscle, walking around with spaghetti arms and legs. Don't follow the lead of those types of people.

You can do conditioning indoors on all pieces of equipment. You can even do it with weights, plyometrics, and even just bodyweight exercises. But I believe the absolute BEST form of conditioning is outdoor sprints on hills, with parachutes, sleds, etc. There are millions of ways of doing conditioning.

High INTENSITY Interval Training(conditioning) is the way to go. Study after study has proven it to be a way more effective form of cardio to burn fat and get you shredded abs. If you increase your training intensity, you increase your results. Now as long as you don't have any limitations, conditioning is the only form of cardio you should be doing. Later on we will discuss how to do some soft tissue work to keep your muscles in check so you can train like a beast seven days a week.

No more being a hamster, be a CHEETAH! Be a LION! Be consistent!

Acceptable times to do LISS

With that said, there are a few acceptable times to do LISS. One is if you are really beat up, sore, and just need to burn more calories to hit your daily calorie burn goal (you'll get yours soon), go for it. As long as its short, occasional, it's no big deal.

If you are taking a day off of training but want to be active, you can do an active recovery day and go do some light LISS to just move the body and get some blood flow or burn a few calories. Also utilize this day to stretch, roll, and work on mobility. (We will discuss that soon)

If you enjoy hiking, biking or other forms of lower intensity activities, go for it. But these do not count as training, nor should they be used as your training. They are extra credit. But keep them to rare minimums. If your spouse or partner wants to go for a hike through the wilderness for some quality time, go for it. If you want to go run some trails once in a while to clear your head or for fun, go for it.

But the bulk of your cardio training, if you choose to do any, should be HIIT conditioning forms. Remember, if your diet is on point and weight training is intense, you won't have to do ANY cardio. But you can add some HIIT to your workout regimen to accelerate your fat loss. We will actually have a weekly "conditioning day" in your training program which you will see soon.

"Energy and persistence conquer all things."
–Benjamin Franklin

Lifts by body part

Want to know what the best exercises are for getting shredded? Want to know what the most effective ones are to develop muscle? Would you like to know how much weight you SHOULD be aiming to lift one day? Well, this is what I'm going to cover in this section.

There are literally thousands of variations of training body parts, but keep in mind that 90% of it is UNNECESSARY crap. You don't need to do the cheesy single arm, single leg, balancing act BS to get shredded. You don't need to hit the body parts from a thousand different angles. The key element to muscle growth and getting shredded are the large compound lifts, the moves that require the recruitment of large muscle groups, and multiple muscle groups to do the work. These are what develop muscle, increase testosterone, growth hormone, and MELT calories.

Isolation movements have their place, but the foundation of our training are the COMPOUND moves: bench, squat, deadlifts, shoulder presses, pull-ups, lunges, etc. These exercises listed below are seriously ALL the moves you will ever need and the basic fundamentals will take you all the way. Sure, later on you can switch some things up to make it more fun or new. But for now, stick to the basics because the basic fundamentals are the foundation of success.

Got it? Okay, good. Now let's talk about the basic moves. With these exercises, I am also going to list the goal weights that you should be aiming to train with for optimal muscular development and results. Keep in mind, I am talking about GOAL weights. Work your way up to these. I'm just giving you an image and target to aim for, because the human mind is a goal-seeking organism. Give it a target and it will pursue it.

These are the Shredded Exec Standards for strength but they only count if you can train with it with control, full range of motion, and good form. So remember, train with your ABILITY, not your ego. Your aim is to be able to train with these weights in the future. The number in the parenthesis is your goal training weight, which is the ideal training weight that you are to set your mind on reaching and surpassing. It will take time to get there so always lift quality reps, good form, and good control.

"Quality over quantity. Always."
–Daymond Sewall

Chest:

Dumbbell Bench Press (120 lb.+)
Dumbbell Bench Incline (100 lb.+)
Dumbbell Fly (60 lb.+)
Dumbbell Fly Incline Bench (50 lb.+)
Barbell Bench Press (225 lb. – twice your bodyweight)
Barbell Bench Press Incline (225 lb.+)
Cable Fly (low, medium, high) (80 lb.+)

Back:

Bent over Barbell Row (225 lb.+)
T-Bar Row (Three 45 lb. plates +)
Single-arm Dumbbell Row (120 lb.+)
Renegade Row (50 lb.+)
Seated Cable Row (250 lb.+)
Seated Lateral Pull Down (200 lb.+)

Pull-ups (Your bodyweight, 20 reps)
Weighted Pull-ups (90 lb.+ strapped)
Chin-ups (Your bodyweight, 20 reps)
Chin-ups (100 lb., strapped)
Close Grip Pull-down (200 lb.+)
Two Arm Dumbbell Row (100 lb.+)

Legs:

Deadlifts (315 lb. – triple your bodyweight)
Barbell Back Squat (225 lb. – twice your bodyweight)
Barbell Split Squat (185 lb. +)
Barbell Walking Lunges (225 lb.+)
Barbell Reverse Lunges (225 lb.+)
Barbell Step Ups (185 lb.+)
Barbell Stiff Leg Deadlift (315 lb.+)
Dumbbell Squat (100s+)
Dumbbell Split Squat (80s+)
Dumbbell Walking Lunges (100s+)
Dumbbell Reverse Lunges (100s+)
Dumbbell Step-ups (80s+)
Dumbbell Stiff leg deadlifts (100s+)
Standing Calf Raises Machine (Entire Stack)
Standing Calf Raises with Dumbbell (100 lb. DB)
Sitting Calf Soleus (Three 45 lb. plates +)

Shoulders:

Barbell Shoulder Press (185 lb.+)
Barbell Front Raise (95 lb.+)
Barbell Rear Deltoid Row (135 lb.+)
Dumbbell Shoulder Press (90 lb.+)

Dumbbell Side Raise (40s+)
Dumbbell Rear Deltoid Fly (30s+)
Dumbbell Front Raise (40s+)
Dumbbell Arnold Press (80s+)
Cable Shoulder Press (120+ depending on machine)
Cable Side Raise (50+ depending on machine)
Cable Rear Delt Fly (40+)
Cable Front Raise (40+)

Triceps:

Barbell Close Grip Bench Press (225 lb.+)
Barbell Skull Crusher (100 lb.+)
Dumbbell Skull Crusher (50s +)
Dumbbell Tri Kickback (40s+)
One Dumbbell Overhead Press (100 lb.+)
V Bar Press-down (120+ depending on machine)
Rope Press-down (80+ depending on machine)
Dips (90 lb+ strapped)
Bodyweight Skull Crusher (your bodyweight, 20 reps)

Biceps:

Barbell Curls (100 lb.+)
Barbell Preacher Curls (100 lb.+)
EZ Bar Curls (110 lb.+)
Dumbbell Curls (50 lb.+)
Seated Concentration Curl (50 lb.+)
Dumbbell Hammer Curls (50 lb.+)
Cable Curl Bar (100 lb.+ depending on machine)

Cable Curl Rope (100 lb.+ depending on machine)

Abs:

Weighted Decline Sit-up (100 lb. DB on chest)
Plank Hold (2 minutes)
Plank Arm Reach (20 times, each side)
Cockroach (30 lb. Dumbbell)
Jackknifes (45 lb.+)
Leg Lifts (10 lb.+)
Reverse Crunches (10 lb.+)
Hanging Knee Raises (20 lb.+)
Hanging Leg lefts (10 lb.+)
Dragon Flag (10 lb. +)
Ab Wheel Rollouts (on toes, face to floor)
Cable Crunch (150 lb.+ depending on machine)
Medicine Ball Plate Crunch (45 lb.+)

Keep in mind these are weight training goals, so some of these weights could take you YEARS to achieve. That's okay; remember that this is a lifestyle. To get the body you want and keep it means LIVING the lifestyle. Training is a PART of life, just like sleeping, eating, and brushing your teeth. Like I said, I'm just giving you GOALS to set the standard of where you SHOULD get to because the human mind is a goal seeking organism.

These exercises are the key staples and literally all the exercises you'll ever need to get shredded and develop a phenomenal physique. Don't overcomplicate it. This process is simply training hard, eating right, and doing both of these consistently week after week after week. You don't need any of the ridiculous stability exercises, the fancy or crazy looking moves.

All you need is to master the basic fundamentals with the key exercises. Fuvk what you read in magazines, or hear on TV. They are usually just selling products, supplements, gadgets, gizmos – all of which you do NOT need. All you need is your macros ON POINT seven days a week, and INTENSE progressive training. Period.

Now that we have the exercises covered, let's talk about HOW we are going to train with them.

HIST (High Intensity Strength Training)

Ready to learn how to train intensely so you don't have to do cardio? Want to learn how to maximize your time in the gym so you get shredded faster?

Remember when I told you that if your diet is on point, that the only form of training that you will ever need to do is intense weight training? HIST is the reason why, because it stands for High Intensity Strength Training. My version of this is basically a type of training that involves lots of supersets, tri-sets or giant sets with a timed rest. This has a very high calorie burn and works on your muscles and your body metabolically. You keep your heart rate elevated, the calories melting, and your body gets shredded, all with just straight LIFTING intensely.

There are many names and acronyms of similar forms of high intensity training with weights. But to simplify it, we will just call it HIST, which is a form of metabolic resistance training. This type of training can be done many ways, but my personal favorite is by doing antagonistic or multiple body parts. This means you train opposing muscle groups, back-to-back in a superset or multiple muscle groups in a tri-set, or giant set fashion.

This is how I train myself to get ready for physique competitions, photoshoots, and how I train my clients to get them ripped and shredded. This method WORKS! (But remember, your diet has to be on point in order for all of this HARD work to pay off.) I have hundreds of different training methods in my arsenal that I use on myself and my clients. But for simplicity and time purposes, I'm going to give you the hacks that are the nuts and bolts that are guaranteed to work. But first, let's talk about some key things you need to know for optimal results.

The connection

"Feel the muscle, and you will reveal more muscle."
–Daymond Sewall

Would you like to get MORE results with the same amount of work? How would you like to get MORE muscular development from your training by using one simple trick each set? When it comes to lifting, what do you think is one of the most vital aspects to muscular development? The weight, the sets, or the reps?

Yes, these are vital components, but the MOST important element of muscular development is your "mind-muscle connection" while lifting those weights, for those reps, and for those sets.

What does this mean? Science (via EMG research) has proven that concentrating on the target muscle results in greater activation of this muscle. This means you need to focus on FEELING the target muscle resisting the weight while lowering, and squeezing the target muscles to lift the weight. It is more than just moving the weight from Point A to Point B. If you focus on feeling the muscle do the work, you will literally get MORE activation out of that muscle, which leads to greater development of that muscle.

Let's take bench press for example, as this is primarily for your chest. As you are lowering the bar, you want to use your pectorals to resist the weight coming down and lower it with control, then at the bottom of the motion, you want to FEEL and squeeze your pecs to press the bar back up. All of this should be done under excellent control. Always make sure you use as heavy of a weight you can handle with good form and good control, feeling your muscles doing the work.

Develop an incredible mind-muscle connection and you will get MORE out of every workout.

Train to gain

"Everybody want to be a bodybuilder,
but don't nobody wanna lift no heavy-ass weights!"
–Ronnie Coleman

Want to know what makes the body develop muscle? Want to know how to develop and maintain it while dieting? When it comes to our training for the first few phases, our number one priority is to increase your output and melt calories, but even though that's our focus, we still train to GAIN. Your mindset and focus is to train to gain muscle.

What does that mean? This means we aren't doing the old-school sissy low weight, high rep BS. This type of thinking comes primarily from body builders who are on cocktails of performance enhancing drugs. As a natural lifter, someone without PED's, lifting low weight and high reps will make you SKINNY.

Light weights have their place. We even have some included in this program, but not as your primary lifts. In order to develop muscle, you must constantly PROGRESSIVELY OVERLOAD your muscles. In order to KEEP the muscle you have gained, you have to keep progressively overloading your muscles, especially while dieting. How do we overload progressively? By constantly pushing the limits on the amount of weight you lift, the reps you squeeze out (with good form on those lifts), or the total volume you do per workout.

For instance, let's say you can bench 225 pounds for five sets of five reps. Progressive overload would be either increasing the reps, adding another set, or adding weight.

- Progressive overload would be doing 225 lb. for 5 sets of 6 reps,
- Or 225 lb. times 6 sets of 5 reps,
- Or adding some weight and doing say 235 lb. times 5 sets of 5 reps.

Any one of these is a form of progressive overload. But the most simple way of doing this is just popping out more reps. So if you feel you have another rep or two in the tank, DO IT. PROGRESSIVELY overload your muscles. Train to gain. If you can do a few sets with two to three more reps, it's time to add some weight to that lift.

So if I am giving you five sets of eight reps, and you bust out a few sets of 11 reps, you need to add some weight. Go up about 5-10 pounds. Muscles will only grow or develop, if they are FORCED to. The are only forced to when OVERLOADED.

"The last three to four reps is what makes the muscles grow. This area of pain divides the champion from someone else who is not a champion."
– Arnold Schwarzenegger

Now know that during the shredding portion of this program, you will build muscle. However, the amount of muscle you will add is in very small doses, but it IS possible to develop muscle during this phase and it will happen.

Want to know why your gains are in small doses? Because muscle growth requires calories. To burn fat and get shredded, we have to be in what caloric state?

Correct: A DEFICIT!

This means your calorie intake is going to be lower. You can and will gain some muscle while shredding; it's just not going to be as significant as when you're shredded and then we start reverse dieting to start focusing on adding size. Once you are shredded, we reverse diet by slowly increasing your calorie intake over time to grow while maintaining your shredded physique. We will discuss that later on. Right now, just focus on getting shredded with a train to gain mentality. Seek the PAIN!

Just know that you ALWAYS lift hard and lift HEAVY like you ARE building. This helps keep your testosterone high, growth hormone production up, and tells your body to keep the muscle it has and it will even add some as needed. So when you train, TRAIN TO GAIN. You do this by focusing on the mind-muscle connection but also training to progressively overload. Focus on getting STRONG. This helps you develop and maintain the muscles you've developed.

Concentrate on every rep of every set, develop the mind-muscle connection, and progressively overload week by week.

"If you train hard, you'll not only be hard, you'll be hard to beat."
–Herschel Walker NFL Champion & MMA Champion

Visualize performance

"Visualize your success, then go and do it!"
-Arnold Schwarzenegger

When you are training, you must visualize your performance. This means visualize you doing the set. Visualize the way you want this muscle to look and the goal result you are training for. You must visualize you HAVING the physique that you are training for. You must go to the gym with the mindset that every single rep you do is getting you closer to that goal. Each rep is going to turn that vision into a reality.

The more focused you are, the more your mind is connected to the muscle and intent on producing that end result, the sooner you will get there.

Seek failure

Don't be afraid to fail and SEEK failure. When it comes to lifting, when it comes to life, we learn the most from our failures. Our failures truly are our lessons and stepping stones to our successes. The same concept applies to business: when we fail and make mistakes, we learn. Those lessons become building blocks to our successes. In the gym, you must push the limits, aim to do more than you think you can do (with good form), push harder than you think you can go. The only way you will ever know that you can squat 315 pounds or deadlift 405 pounds is if you are willing to fail.

If you are afraid of failure, then you will never grow. Never grow muscle, never grow as an executive, and never grow as a person. So don't be afraid to fail. Failure is part of success, it is WHY you will have successes in your life. This principle can be applied to everything in life.

"How you do one thing is how you do anything."

-Unknown

The discipline, effort, consistency, focus, and work ethic you put forth in the gym is exactly what you do in all areas of life. If you quit when it gets hard, when it burns, when it's challenging, or only train when it is easy and convenient, this is what you do in all areas of life. In life you are probably only doing what is easy, what is convenient, and you avoid the challenging things, or quit when things get hard. I am a firm believer in this quote, and have found it to be VERY, very true in almost every person I have ever met.

So by developing the discipline, conditioning your mind to achieve everything that you want to achieve in the gym, with your body, training daily, completing your workouts, achieving your small daily training goals, this also trains your subconscious mind. This literally sends a message to your subconscious mind that *"I am committed. I am dedicated. I always do what I intend to do. I am disciplined. I will do whatever it takes. I am successful."*

Your subconscious is what controls up to 98% of your daily behaviors, actions, decisions, habits, choices. So if you are training your subconscious to believe *"I am committed. I am dedicated. I always do what I intend to do. I am disciplined. I will do whatever it takes. I am successful"*, what do you think your body is going to look like? Incredible, huh?

What do you think your business is going to look like?

Awesome, huh?

How do you think your relationships are going to improve? Drastically, huh?

What do you think your income is going to look like?

AMAZING, huh?

Remember in the beginning of the book when I told you that this is going to completely transform your life? This is why. What you establish on the inside with your mind and within the gym, you will also accomplish on the outside. Success on the inside leads to success on the outside.

"What you do in the gym, you do in life.
How you do one thing is how you do everything."
-Daymond Sewall

"STFU and train!"
–Unknown

When we train, we train with the train to gain mentality and progressively overload the muscle, this mentality is primarily to just help you maintain the muscle you have while dieting. But we also take this to another level, we also train with the intent to melt fat. When we train, when we lift, we save time, maximize your calorie output, and get the most out of your workout by training at a high intensity. We do that by using a form of training known as High Intensity Strength Training.

We do this by training multiple muscle groups per set. This means we don't do the old 3x10, just do one set then rest for 3 minutes like the average gym goer. We increase the intensity, increase your heart rate and calorie burn by training two to three exercises per set, performed back-to-back. Then we rest for a short, specific amount of time and repeat for the desired amount of sets.

We do this to increase the intensity, burn more calories, and maximize your time in the gym. There is no time for BS, no time for playing on your phone, and no time for watching TV. You are in the gym for one reason and one reason only.

What is that reason? That reason is to MAKE progress and get shredded, so we train HARD and INTENSE.

An example of HIST is doing supersets of opposing muscles. One muscle group recovers while the other is getting blasted, and you take a short rest or zero rest and start the next set. You can get MORE done within a short amount of time, melt calories, increase your metabolism, and get your body shredded. This is HOW we are able to get shredded without doing frickin' cardio. Fuvk cardio! Arnold Schwarzenegger used to train in a very similar fashion.

Here is an example of a HIST workout for the

Shredded Exec Training Phase #1 - Chest and Back

SuperSet #1

Performed back to back, then rest 60, and repeat for 4 sets. (4 sets of 10 reps)

A1. Dumbbell Single Arm Row 10 reps each side
A2. Barbell Bench Press 10 reps
Rest 60. Repeat for total of 4 sets.

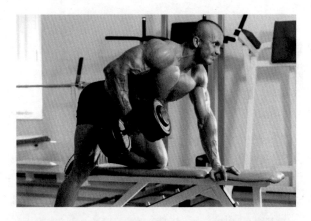

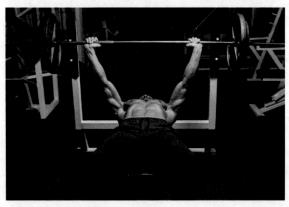

In this example, you are doing two exercises per set. You start with Single Arm Dumbbell Row for 10 reps on each side, then straight to Barbell Bench for 10 reps heavy, Rest 60 seconds. Then repeat for total of four sets.

In our training we will be doing three or more supersets per workout daily. So after completing all four sets of A1-A2, you then move to B1-B2, then C1-C2. Then you're done. You will find that this type of training will have you huffing and puffing, and maybe even looking for a trashcan to puke in. It will keep you focused, training hard, burning calories, and save you TIME. There's no time for chit-chat or BS. You are there to TRAIN.

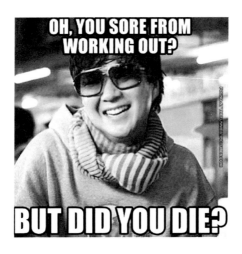

There are a million ways of doing this, but that's a simple example of how we train. Do this the correct way with heavy, challenging weights, an awesome form, timed rest periods, intense effort, and you will NEVER have to step foot on a cardio machine again if you don't want to. This is the secret to how we get shredded by primarily pure lifting.

I personally LOVE doing sprints, parachutes, sleds, stadiums, and do it once a week for fun and conditioning. We also have one day a week where we do conditioning in the program so you can accelerate your fitness levels, increase your work capacity, improve your recovery ability, and to get shredded. You will look like a GOD, be shredded, and have incredible health.

Our training protocol has you lifting five days, conditioning on the sixth, with flexibility and prehab on the seventh day.

Did you notice I have you training seven days a week?

That's intentional. You need to develop the habit of going more often so you can achieve your goal quicker. This also sends a message to your subconscious that you are committed, consistent, persistent, do whatever it takes, dedicated, disciplined and do what you intend to do. This will transfer to your behaviors, choices, and actions in business. So even on a day that you intend to rest, go in and train your flexibility and mobility. Stretch, foam roll muscles, sauna, or whatever you like, but you must train your body in some way seven days a week.

Heart rate training

When we train, we train to what? Yes, to progressively overload. To develop and maintain muscle. To improve strength. To burn calories and melt fat so we get shredded.

How do you know how hard you are working? How many calories you burned? How do you know what your average heart rate or max heart rate is? By using a heart rate monitor! One of the methods that we use to increase your EFFORT is through Heart Rate Training. The higher you keep your heart rate during training, the more calories you burn.

The more calories you burn, the more you...?

Lose!

We use this tool as constant feedback, as a guide, and as a GOAL to make us work HARDER. What happens when we work harder? Yes, we get results FASTER.

This simply means we wear a heart rate monitor to constantly watch your heart rate and we aim for a specific heart rate minimum and a specific calorie burn goal per day. The heart rate monitor I am going to recommend tells you your heart rate, your heart rate average and peak, and your calories burned.

You will find that when you start wearing this your training goes to another level! I personally cannot even workout without mine. I have a few that I keep in my gym bag for backups or for different types of training. But you only need one, and that one is the one I have below. So depending on your size and weight, your calorie burn goals will vary.

Here is a simple rule of thumb for Heart Rate Training while lifting and conditioning:

1. 100 BPM while lifting

When you are lifting, your goal is to keep your heart rate above 100 BPM. When your training has started (excluding warm-up), your goal is to keep your heart rate above 100 BPM at a minimum. The higher your average during training, the more your body is burning. So if you are resting between sets for 60 seconds and at 45 seconds in your heart rate drops to 100, start your next set NOW to keep it up! We want to keep your heart rate up so we keep your heart rate average and calorie output HIGH.

Your heart rate monitor will give you a report when your workout is over, telling you your average and maximum heart rate for the workout. You want to have a HIGH average heart rate, we do this by keeping your heart rate up by never letting it go below a 100 and training hard with short rests.

On a typical day of lifting, your heart rate report may look like "Average 120 BPM, Maximum 165 BPM," but an OUTSTANDING day would like "Average 135+ BPM, Maximum 185+ BPM." This would be an excellent effort day! We use this tool to push you and increase intensity so you BURN more calories per workout. Training at a high intensity burns more calories DURING the workout and creates more of an afterburn effect, so your metabolism is stoked for hours after your training is over.

2. The 180 Rule of Conditioning

"If you're not peaking 180, you're not pushing your limits.
Push harder!"
–Daymond Sewall

This primarily applies to your conditioning training when you do your high intensity interval training, but it's a good standard to assess how hard you're really working during lifting too. What this means is when you are doing your sprint intervals, your goal is to peak over 180 BPM a few times throughout your workout. You're not really WORKING until you peak 180 BPM, in my opinion. Doesn't matter who you are, what age, what shape you're in; that's the standard. When doing HIIT, your goal is to peak it on your high interval, but sometimes it may take you a few intervals to hit 180 BPM.

The rule of 180 BPM is the level of effort I expect and you should aim for. The more out of shape you are, the faster heart rate rises and slower it lowers. The more in shape you are, the

HARDER you have to work to get there. Yes, you can hit 180. If you haven't before, it's because you just haven't ever pushed your body hard enough to see it. You won't die, although you may feel like it. The worst thing that will happen is you get exhausted and stop. But that would be what? Failure! We seek failure, remember? We PUSH limits. Just make sure you have a clean bill of health from your doctor before you live by this rule.

If you are really out of shape, you may hit 180+ easily and your heart rate stays higher longer because your recovery ability is poor. Someone terribly out of shape may be hitting over 180 just doing very basic exercises with minimal or no weight. As they stay consistent, their body will progress and they will have to work harder to hit this standard.

If you are fit or have a history of doing lots of cardio (distance running, cycling, triathlons), your cardio capacity is going to be greater, so it is going to be much, much more strenuous to hit the 180 BPM mark. But it CAN be done. You are used to pacing yourself, so that is over. It's time to PUSH yourself! The 180 rule always stands. This is how you continually push your limits.

I have a resting heart rate of about 39-45 BPM average (depending on time of year and training) and even I get mine up to 185-200+ when I do my conditioning workouts. That is an INSANE accomplishment and if I can get mine that high, you can too.

"It's your mind quitting, not your body. Suck it up and push it!"
–Daymond Sewall

It can be done. It's your MIND that's wanting to quit, not your body. You CAN hit it. So DTFW and get it!

3. Hit your Calorie Burn Goal DAILY.

We use your heart rate monitor to give you instant feedback on your effort and to give you a calorie burn GOAL. You're in the gym to complete each workout and to burn a specific amount of calories daily. Your heart rate monitor is your tool that is going to give you instant feedback to how hard you're working and how many calories you've burned based off of your effort.

This means you don't get to leave the gym or lay your head on your pillow until your WORK is put in for the day. I don't care if you have to split it up into two or three workouts because you are busy one day and have appointments that don't allow you to get it in one workout. Hit your calorie burn goal DAILY. You don't deserve to leave the gym or sleep until you do. Period. DTFW!

Here is the list of calorie burn goals. The heavier you are, the MORE you need to burn. So if you are heavier, aim for the HIGH number. Remember, these are minimums. If you want faster results, do MORE than what is required. So even though I say to burn 700 calories minimum, if you are burning a minimum of 1,000+ calories, you are going to get shredded faster.

5'6" and Below 500-700+
5'7" - 5'10" and 700-1,000+
5'11" and over 1,000-1,500+

That is your calorie burn goal you need to invest DAILY.

So what were those 3 rules again?

1. 100 BPM minimum while lifting. Keep your average high.
2. 180 BPM, peaking during HIIT training.
3. Hit your calorie burn goal DAILY.

Two tools to elevate your results

These are the two tools that we use to elevate and expedite your results. We want that, right? Yes or yes? So go online and order one of these.

1. Heart Rate Monitor. (Polar FT60, A300, or M400).

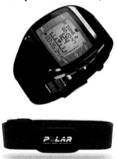

Once you train with a HRM you will never want to train without it.

2.   Workout journal

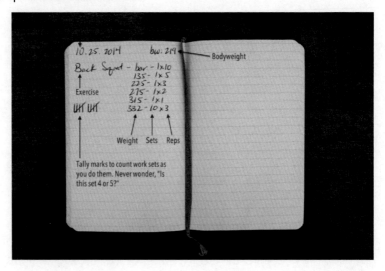

Just like how you plan your business day, to-do lists, and important tasks, you need to be doing the same thing for your training. You NEED to write down the workout you plan to do and keep track of the weights, sets, reps. Your goal is to BEAT what you did last workout. So if you did a Dumbbell Bench Press with 80 pounds x eight reps last time, this time the goal is to progressively overload and get nine or more reps or if you feel strong enough, bump it up to 85 pounds.

The intent is to always try to progressively overload your muscles week by week. This is HOW you continue to make progress, add muscle, and keep your results coming. The only way you'll remember what you did is if you have a record of what you did. The only way you'll have a goal to accomplish is if you have a written record of last workout's performance.

Remember, the human mind is a goal-seeking organism, so it will try to achieve whatever target you set. The only way you know the target is if you have it in writing and focus on beating it. So invest in a notebook and plan your workouts and aim to beat what you did last time. This is how the greats became the greats. Just like how you track expenses, income, sales, and appointments, to succeed in business, you need to track your training to succeed in getting shredded.

"All winners are trackers."
-Darren Hardy

Train with your ability

"Ego lifters are insecure 'lil bitches."
–Daymond Sewall

You need to be progressively overloading and pushing your body beyond its limits. But with that said, train with your ABILITY. This means you don't go in the gym and "ego lift." Ego lifting is like that guy that stacks tons of plates on a bar, then precedes to look like an idiot doing quarter reps. The guy who puts three or four plates each side on a squat bar, and barely bends his knees in an attempt to squat, but really only looks like he's having a seizure. DON'T be that guy. Yes, you need to lift hard and heavy, but you have to lift with your ABILITY. You're not going to be able to lift that heavy yet. One day with time, effort, and consistency, you will.

What does that mean?

That means FULL range of motion, good form, and good control. This is technically sound training. NO ego lifting. As you keep training hard and consistently, your strength levels will get there and you will be able to have some awesome lifts that feed the ego. That comes with TIME. But don't go in the gym to impress anybody. Train and always lift with your ability.

But with that said, don't be a pussy, push your limits, make sure you BEAT what you did last week by doing one more rep or a little more weight, forcing your body to progress to the next level. Are you going to have bad days? Absolutely. Do your best. Are you going to have days where you can't beat last week? Absolutely. Do your best and try to beat it next week.

"Train with your ability and you will become shredded and sexy."
-Daymond Sewall

Shredded Exec Training Phases

Are you ready to learn how to put this all together and start training like a beast? Are you ready to take your body, mind, aesthetics to another level? Are you ready to get shredded? Let's do this!

This program is set up in three phases: SET Phase 1, 2, and 3. Each phase is set up to prep you for the intensity of the next. All three are very challenging and are going to get you shredded. In Phase 1, we are doing supersets of opposing muscle groups. In Phase 2 we do a tri-set. It's basically a superset like Phase 1, but with another exercise added to the set, making it a tri-set (tri = 3). Then in Phase 3, we go back to two moves per set, but stepping up the intensity of each set by adding extreme stimulation training.

It will look like this:
Phase 1: Supersets + 1 day of HIIT conditioning
Phase 2: Tri-sets + 1 day of HIIT conditioning
Phase 3: Extreme Stimulation Training(Shred Style), SD20 Method

Extreme Stimulation Training (Shred Style)

This program is set up in phases to progress you as your body progresses. One of the methods we use in Phase 3 of this program is a form of High Intensity Strength Training, just with EXTREME stimulation. There are literally millions of ways of doing this and hundreds of different "stimulation" methods.

But for simplicity, I'm going to give you one of my favorites, which is the SD20 Method for Phase 3. This SINGLE method is a game changer and is very, very effective. I personally use this method to get shredded as I get closer to shows and photoshoots. This is why I'm giving you my secret weapon here in Phase 3.

So what is Extreme Stimulation Training? Let's call it training beyond failure. You see, the typical theory of training to failure is doing a lift where you could not possibly lift one more rep and actually need help getting the weight up. Let's say you're doing squats 225 pounds and you had to be spotted to hit the eighth rep because you couldn't complete it alone.

You hit failure, right? But is it possible you could drop the weight to 185 pounds and squat some more reps? Then when you fail at that weight, you could drop to 135 pounds and do a few more reps, right? The answer is YES to all of the above.

This means that instead of just hitting failure at 225 pounds for 8 reps, you hit failure two more times with two more weights, getting triple the failure. Do you see how EXTREME this is? Do you see how much more progress you will get from pushing your limits like this? This set is going to feel like you are crawling through HELL, screaming, sweat pouring off your face, and pain searing from the burning in your quads. Your heart rate is going to skyrocket, your calorie output go through the roof, and your muscle development get stimulated. This is how you are going to get the best results, this is called Extreme Stimulation Training.

It's frickin' awesome! This is an example of Extreme Stimulation Training, but you have to wait until you get to Phase 3 to do this. Phases 1 and 2 are prepping you for this type of training, so make sure you follow the course.

Examples of E.S.T.

> ***"Unless you puke, faint, or die, KEEP GOING!"***
> ***–Jillian Michaels***

We will be using SD20 method for our Phase 3, but here are some other examples of Extreme Stimulation Training.

Drop Set- When you cannot complete another rep on your own with the weight you are using, reduce the weight, pump out a few more reps until you fail, and then reduce the weight again and pump out more reps. You can do this for three, four, or more drops. I personally am a fan of three total subsets.

Negatives- Using heavier weight than you can truly lift, lower the weight super slow for 4-10 seconds, then have a partner help you lift. You are essentially just resisting the weight as its lowering (negative) but your partner helps you lift.

Rest Pause- Pick a desired number of reps (10-40), but using a weight that's your 3-8 rep max to achieve it. For instance, let's say your goal is 20 reps, you choose a weight you can only do 5 reps max, do 5 reps, REST 20 seconds, then do a couple more. Rest again and repeat until you hit a total of 20 reps. It may look like 5 reps, 2, 1, 2, 3, 1, 3, 2,1 to complete one set of 20. Basically it took 9 mini sets to complete that 20 rep set of Rest Pause method. This is an example of a 20 rep rest pause technique. It's gnarly! You can do the same with any rep range. 40 Method using your 8 rep max weight, with 45 seconds rest is another one of my favs. Use these when you want to mix things up, or are crunched for time. Make sure you have a spotter or use machines or dumbbells so you don't get stuck under a barbell.

Top Halves- This technique is used when you hit failure with a weight, then you do 3-5 more half reps from the top to stimulate the muscle more. For instance, let's say you're benching 225 lb. for 8 reps, you fail at the eighth, then you do half reps from the top half way down and back up 5 five times to finish off that set. You will need a spotter for if you're using a barbell, so I'd recommend only using this with dumbbells or machines if you don't have a partner.

SD20(Phase #3 choice) – This is the one we are using for Phase 3. This is a form of a drop set, but with a rep range GOAL and with the focus on the initial super heavy weight. Each set is 20 reps, but we achieve this by doing 3 reps HEAVY, 7 reps HEAVY, then 10 reps medium heavy. The most important weights are the 3 and 7 rep weights.

Start with your 3 rep max weight you can do with flawless form and great control. Then the heaviest weight you can rep for 7 reps to kill it some more. Then the 10 reps as heavy as possible, but light enough you can do all 10 with good form. These last 10 reps, focus on the form and technique and a deep mind-muscle connection, FEELING your muscles lift and lower the weight. This method is going to skyrocket your heart rate, melt calories, and kick your ass.

For instance, let's say you're doing Single Arm Dumbbell Row. You would do 120 lb. x 3 reps, 90 lb. x 7 reps, then 60 lb. x 10 to finish it. Then switch sides. Then move to the other move/moves paired with this and repeat the method. This is a BEAST! Now you see why it's Phase 3 and why we don't do cardio. Your heart rate will go through the roof during this type of training. My heart rate usually peaks over 180 BPM when I do this method with single arm rows.

The reason why we are using the SD20 style is for two main reasons: it hits the HEAVY lifts for strength and hypertrophy, and will absolutely elevate your heart rate and melt calories – all in one set. It's very intense, but highly EFFECTIVE and fun.

There are just a few examples of EST (Extreme Stimulation Training). There are lots of ways of doing this, but for simplicity and effectiveness, we are using a prescribed system that is guaranteed to work if done correctly. So follow the phases as directed because each one is preparing you for the next one. This is a SYSTEM, so follow the system and you will get the results.

All you have to do is what? DO THE FUVKING WORK!

An example of this would look like this for working the chest and back:

Warm-up
50 Pushups
50 DB Bent Over Row (2 DBs)
Rest 2 minutes

Shred Style Set #1. DB Bench/DB Row
Motion Warm-up DB Bench Press 20 reps, 10 reps
Motion Warm-up DB Row 20 reps, 10 reps

DB Bench SD20

120x3, 90x7, 60x10 reps

DB Single Arm Row SD20

120x3, 90x7, 60x10

Rest 60 seconds

Do 4 sets

Shred Style Set #2. **DB Incline Bench/Weighted Chin-ups**

Motion Warm-up Incline Bench 20 reps

Motion Warm-up Chin-ups 20 reps

DB incline Bench SD20

100x3, 80x7, 60x10

Weighted Chin-ups

90x3, 45x7, bodyweight x10

Rest 60-120 seconds

Do 4 sets

Shred style Set #3. DB Chest Fly to Wide Lat Pulldown

Motion Warm-up DB Fly 25x20

Motion Warm-up Wide Lat Pull 100x20

DB Fly SD20

60x3, 45x7, 30x10

Wide Lat Pulldown

200x3, 160x7, 120x10

Always make sure you do a very thorough warm-up, take as many sets as you need to fill the muscles with blood. So do a few sets of warm-ups, working your way up to your working weights. Start with like 50% your max, then 60%, then 80%. You'll notice I put a "Motion Warm-up" at the beginning of every set. Make sure you DO THESE to prep your muscles for this specific motion. This will help you lift heavier, have better mind-muscle connection, and keep you SAFE. Staying injury free is KEY to being able to train like a beast yearly.

Like I said in the beginning, there are millions of ways of doing this. Phase 3 isn't for sissies, beginners, or intermediates; it's more for advanced lifters. So stay in Phase 2 as long as you feel you need before moving to Phase 3. Also, when you first move to Phase 3, you may only be able to do three sets of the SD20 instead of the recommended four. As you progress, you can add in the fourth.

Like I keep saying, there are a million ways of training. I'm giving you a specific program guaranteed to work if done correctly to simplify your life and cut through all the confusion. This system WORKS. I use it on clients to get them shredded, I use it myself to get shredded. Just like there are a million ways of training, there are a million ways of doing a workout split. But just to give you a rigid guideline, here is what our split is going to look like for your S.E.T. program.

Training Schedule.
Day 1: Legs/Abs
Day 2: Back/Chest
Day 3: Shoulders
Day 4: Legs/Calves
Day 5: Biceps/Triceps
Day 6: Shred Conditioning
Day 7: Flexibility/Mobility/Prehab

This training program is designed for MAXIMUM results, and is very, very intense. It is going to get you shredded and will get you in the BEST shape of your life, both mentally and physically. Your muscle groups are set up in this order for a reason, we train the major body parts such as legs, back, chest the first two days while you are fresh. These are the MOST important body parts not only for looks, but for calorie burn, growth, and hormone production. Then I will give you some active recovery and you'll be training your polishing muscles such as abs and calves on Day 3.

Then it's back to work on Days 4 and 5 on the aesthetics, hitting shoulders, biceps, and triceps. Day 6 is shred conditioning, a pure fat burning day, to work on your shreds and improve your health and work capacity. Then Day 7 is a flexibility, mobility, and prehab day. This is time you MUST invest in doing foam rolling, soft tissue work, and stretching to keep your muscles in check so you can perform your BEST next week on Days 1-6. So Make sure that you invest a lot of time into your flexibility, mobility, prehab so that way you can train at 100% effort consistently. We will discuss that more in detail later. Like I said, this is a system! Follow it, do as directed, and you will look, feel, and perform better than you EVER expected.

So there you go. that's how you get a six-pack without doing any boring cardio. Be CONSISTENT.

Review:

Let's Review:

1. What kind of cardio do we avoid?
2. What is the only kind of cardio we do?
3. What is HIIT? What is an easy example?
4. What are some of the benefits of HIIT training?
5. What are the only times doing LISS is acceptable?
6. How do we get shredded without doing any cardio?
7. What's the ONLY kind of cardio you should do?

8. How many days should you be in the gym?
9. What is HIST?
10. How many phases are there in the Shred Exec Training
11. Program? What two tools do you need to take your training to the next level?
12. Get a notebook to track training. Sets, reps, and weights, and beat what you did last week.
13. What's the 100 rule? What's the 180 rule?
14. What is the EST (ShredStyle) training method we are using in Phase #3?

"The vision of a champion is someone who is bent over, drenched in sweat, and to the point of exhaustion, when no one else is watching."
–Anson Dorrance (Coach of Mia Hamm)

[11]

Prehab

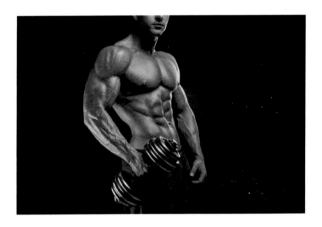

What's the most common reason for someone to stop training, or avoid training certain exercises? INJURIES! PAIN! How do we avoid injuries and pain? PREHAB!

WTF is prehab?!

Prehab means exactly that: PREHAB. This means we do a lot of mobility work, rolling, and stretching to keep your muscles in check so we can train like a beast and stay injury free. We PREhab so we don't have to Rehab you from you developing an injury. Along with keeping you injury free, having more flexibility and mobility leads to more strength, greater muscle gains, and fuller, thicker muscles.

Mobility is how a joint moves, while flexibility is the length of a muscle. Think of mobility as an umbrella covering a range of factors that affect the range of motion around a joint. One of these components is flexibility; it's difficult to move a joint if the connected muscles around it don't stretch far enough to allow it.

Why are these important? Good question. Simply put, if you have muscles that are tight or imbalanced, it will directly prevent the optimal recruitment of the muscle you are training, affects the muscles being recruited, and leads to compensations and eventually pain or injury.

For instance, let's take tight chest (pectorals). This is a very common imbalance due to hours spent sitting or being behind a computer for most Americans. It's also one of the primary causes of terrible posture and shoulder issues. I personally used to have really tight pecs, which led to 17 shoulder dislocations on my left side and five dislocations on my right. Talk about PAIN!!!! Obviously, this was YEARS ago, way before I learned all this incredible information and my shoulders are awesome now. Zero surgeries. Zero Pain. I train like a beast year-round now.

My point is that I know firsthand how BAD it can be if you neglect your flexibility and mobility. I know most of you neglect it now as well, so it's very common. This is why I have added this section to the book.

Would you like to know how injuries happen? Let's take tight pecs for an example. When your chest gets tight, your shoulders are pulled forward (protracted), shortening your pecs. The pecs are shortened (tight and smaller), which causes your shoulders to be misaligned. What do you think happens when you train chest? Due to the imbalance, your chest cannot stretch or contract with its full potential to produce force. It limits your range of motion and your chest is not working at its optimal level, meaning it's weaker.

So if your chest is weaker, cannot produce the strength that it needs to, and your shoulders are rounded forward, what do you think is doing the work when you do bench press or any form of chest exercise?

Your deltoids! Your delts (shoulders) overcompensate and become the prime mover. They become the primary muscle moving the weight and the primary muscles that get the training. Ever see the guy with big shoulders, yet a smaller/nonexistent chest? I call these guys "Captain Protraction" from his protracted shoulders. He's been training with tight pecs for years, overdeveloping his delts and undertraining his chest. So he has well-developed or overdeveloped delts and an underdeveloped chest. This will also eventually lead to a shoulder injury.

We want big developed pecs, right? So what do you think we need to do with your chest? Keep it loose and increase the mobility of it, right or right? But wait, that's not all. Having tight pecs not only affects your chest development, but it inhibits your back from getting properly developed as well.

Because of the forward position of the shoulders, it reduces the range of motion and activation of the back musculature, limiting its development when training the back as well. This leads to MORE compensations, more altered joint motion, and eventually could lead to a shoulder injury. But wait, that's not all. Having tight pecs also affects your shoulder training. It prevents the proper range of motion for overhead pressing movements and restricts motion for all the other shoulder movements.

All these compensations and imbalances also lead to knots in your traps, which are PAINFUL and shoulder joint injuries. Sounds terrible, huh? Wait, there's more!

Another common one is tight calves, when your calves are tight it prevents you from being able to squat deep, bend over, or deadlift properly due to the limited ankle mobility. When you bend your knees to squat or deadlift, your ankle has limited mobility and this leads to compensations, more stress on the Achilles tendon, knees, back, and even affects the shoulders. Having tight calves could lead to a shoulder injury as well, due to the compensations at the hip which affect your pelvis, which your lats attach to. Your lats attach to your upper arm, which affects your shoulder mobility.

Sucks, huh!? So as you can see, it not only prevents the development of the target muscle, it affects many other muscles development as well. It's a domino effect of compensations and altered motion that lead to underdeveloped target muscle or joint/muscle injuries.

Now do you see why having good flexibility and mobility is crucial to your success? Now do you see why I have included this in this book for you? I want you shredded, rich, healthy and performing like a BEAST year-round. This is why taking care of your flexibility and mobility is very, very important.

Want to know what the most common imbalances are? The most common problem areas are the chest, lats, hip flexors, IT bands, quads, and calves. These lead to shoulder injuries, low back pain, knee pain, and knotted trap issues that are excruciating.

How to stay injury free

What's the number one way to staying injury-free? To keep your diet CLEAN, by eating a whole food anti-inflammatory diet. This means avoiding ALL processed foods, ALWAYS. Foods that are manmade, contain flour, sugar, chemicals, and processed oils set you up for injury and pain.

Why? Good question. These foods are highly inflammatory to our bodies. When you eat an inflammatory food, it will always inflame and flare up pain in an area with a preexisting issue. This means an old injury, a knotted muscle, a recently trained sore muscle, or a tight area. Think about the last time you had back pain, knee pain, shoulder pain, or just felt really tight and your workout was hindered. You probably just associated it with age but that's NOT the case at all.

Think about the foods you ate within the week prior, I guarantee you if you think back, you will find you ate something processed one to seven days prior. That's not a coincidence, that's called systemic inflammation. It happens to ALL of us if we eat something inflammatory. Most people just don't realize it because most people don't train and they don't use their muscles often, so they don't notice the inflammation as much. But get them working out and BAM! PAIN! They always want to blame getting older, but that's not the cause. The cause is called systemic inflammation.

Making a poor food choices is the cause and it will usually always lead to aches, pain, joint issues, pulled muscles, and your training will be set back. Especially foods containing the triple or quadruple whammies (sugar, flour, processed oils, dairy) like bread, pasta, pizza, donuts, cakes, cookies, etc. If you have ONE bite of these, PAIN is guaranteed. Those are some of the most injurious foods. The inflammation can last for 7-14 days after eaten, too. It's not worth it.

But like most people, you will probably have to learn the hard way and it will take an injury before you believe what I just said.

"A smart man makes a mistake, learns from it, and never makes that mistake again. But a wise man finds a smart man, learns from him how to avoid the mistake altogether."
-Roy H. Williams

So if you don't believe me, go eat pizza, bread, and pasta on Saturday, then go train legs on Monday and watch how terrible you feel. Watch how tight your body feels and how your muscles and/or joints ache. Watch how your knees or back hurts or how your quads or hamstrings hurt. That's IF you're able to even get to the gym, because these foods also slow blood flow to the brain, making you lazy, lethargic and have brain fog. So you may feel like such shit you won't even want to train. But you have to suck it up and go anyway so you can learn this lesson!

This is a scientifically proven fact. Either be wise and learn from what I'm teaching you, or you go make the mistake and learn your own lesson.

My inflammation story

Let me give you a quick story. Years ago before I really knew how much processed foods and certain ingredients really affected the body, I used to do a weekly cheat meal. Usually on Saturday, I would go to a restaurant and have a little of whatever I wanted. These foods usually were processed and sometimes contained flour and sugar, which you know now are TERRIBLE for your system. One time on one of these cheat days, I had a little cake, a couple slices of pizza, and some other processed foods.

The VERY next day I went to a local football field and was about to do some conditioning. I was feeling rather sluggish and really tight, but just pushed through it and knew that once I got warmed up, I'd feel better. I did a few warm-up light sprints, then as I started to increase my warm-up speed, POP! I partially tore/pulled my right hamstring!

I was on the ground in searing pain with tears in my eyes. I knew EXACTLY what it was: the flour and processed foods from my meal the day prior. The inflammation was so high that it made me super, super tight and inflamed. The already tight and knotted part of my hammy, combined with the tension, caused it to partially tear and pull. This was awful pain.

I got up and hobbled home and started doing some rehab to loosen it. It took months for me to be 100% again. I couldn't straighten my leg fully for almost THREE MONTHS. I hobbled around, couldn't lift as heavy on a lot of my moves, had to modify my leg training, and it completely affected ALL of my training for that entire time. Needless to say, it fuvking sucked. I vowed from that moment on that I would NEVER, EVER touch anything with flour, processed foods, or those that could possibly contain flour EVER AGAIN. I say flour because it is the absolute WORST.

My discovery

What was really awesome was about two weeks after I made this commitment, all the little random aches and tightness I used to have here and there completely DISAPPEARED. I have an old motocross injury that has always caused pain for YEARS – GONE. I had a triceps issue that used to bug me on my left arm – GONE. My muscle tightness I was just used to because I thought it was normal – GONE!

All these years, all the issues and aches I had were all caused from that ONE fuvking cheat meal I had on Saturdays. WOW! After I started feeling so good, I WAS SOLD!!! No more processed foods for me EVER, especially anything that has flour like bread, pizza, pasta, cakes, cookies, etc.

You can do a little test yourself or you can just be wise and learn from OTHER people's mistakes. If you're one of the smart ones that prefers to learn from other people's mistakes and lessons, then just follow the rules of EAT REAL FOOD ONLY. Keep your diet clean and you will live lean and perform like a BEAST. Always. Either way you will learn, and agree that keeping your diet clean is key to staying injury-free and a becoming a shredded beast.

Post-training stretch

The other way to always stay injury-free is to ALWAYS stretch the muscles you used AFTER you train them. Do this to relax and turn off the muscles. Otherwise, they will tighten up, alter joint motion, and eventually lead to pain or an injury. Always stretch after you train. Never just walk out of the gym without stretching, because this should always be the last thing you do before you go home.

Soft tissue work

To improve to mobility of your joints and increase blood flow to muscles, making them fuller and bigger in appearance, you have to do frequent soft tissue work. This includes rolling (self myofascial release), and/or muscle scraping to break up the adhesions and scar tissue that will develop in ALL muscles. This will improve your ability to increase flexibility and improve all joint mobility.

Rolling

Rolling is what is referred to as SMFR (self myofascial release). This used to be called "foam rolling" but over the past decade, TONS of different products have hit the market that are NOT foam that you can now roll on. From pipes, hard rubber, metal, balls, plastic, all with the same purpose to break up tight muscles and knots, relieve soreness and increase joint mobility. Rolling is one of the KEYS to staying injury-free.

I recommend getting four tools to carry in your gym bag at all times. These tools will save you thousands of dollars in trips to the doctor from an injury and save you from losing any time training.

Mobility stick and cradle on www.RogueFitness.com

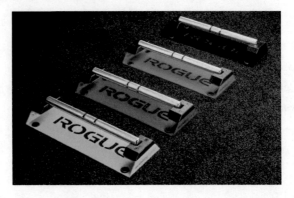

The Supernova 80mm found on www.RogueFitness.com

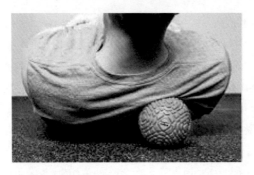 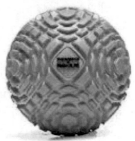

Muscle scraping

Another way of increasing blood flow, mobility, fixing an injury, and preventing injury is muscle scraping. Muscle scraping has a few names, such as the Graston technique, Guasha (Chinese method), and IASTM (instrument assisted soft tissue mobilization), to name a few. This is a secret of mine that only elite chiropractors, massage therapists, physical therapists, and great trainers utilize to fix their clients' mobility issues. Muscle scraping is similar in theory to rolling in the fact that your goal is to break up knotted muscles and increase mobility.

But muscle scraping also breaks down scar tissue, fascia restrictions, and you can address the muscles, tendons, and some ligaments of the joint. Muscle scraping is also a much FASTER treatment, is more aggressive, and very, effective. You can literally fix an issue within seconds. However, it is very painful and it can leave you with some serious bruising the first time that an area gets scraped. So what? If you bruise, it heals, but the pain is eliminated if done correctly.

Personally, I keep lots of these tools on hand in my gym and workout bag. I have even been known to give them to clients as presents. I recommend the tool below called the Mobility Star, and you can find it on www.RogueFitness.com.

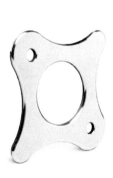 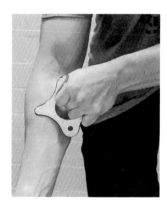

How to do muscle scraping is very simple. Just grab a tool and lube the area you intend to treat (with coconut oil). With firm pressure, scrape the tool up and down the muscle. You will feel bumps, cracks, lumps, pain, and immediately notice blood rushing to the area, turning your skin red.

You want to break up all those adhesions, knotted tissues, aches, and painful areas. So keep scraping until the pain dissipates. As the pain starts to reduce, push deeper into the tissue. It's always better if someone else does this for you, or a certified Graston or IASTM practitioner. But you CAN do it yourself. Just look up IASTM or Graston on YouTube. It is very commonsense technique.

I also recommend this tool for your calves, quads, Zuka4 handlebar. www.ZukaTools.com.

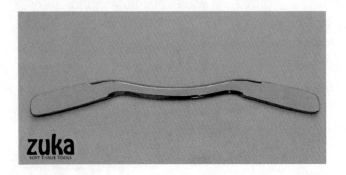

I recommend using rolling and muscle scraping DAILY to keep your muscles looking and feeling their best. Like I said, keep those tools in your gym bag and if you ever feel something is tight, knotted, or achy, use one of those tools to fix it and keep training. I also keep some in my shower to do at home in the evening. This is very easy to do when you are soapy and is a great habit to establish.

We covered how to fix yourself, so let's talk about having someone else fix you.

Massage

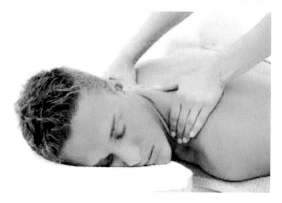

The other way of staying injury free is to schedule a deep tissue or sports massage every one to two weeks. The training you are going to be going through is TOUGH and you are going to need a lot of maintenance to keep up. The work you do on yourself will be sufficient, but it's ALWAYS more beneficial and effective when someone else is doing it. They will also hit areas you don't know about or cannot reach well. I recommend either finding a massage therapist that knows about muscle scraping or introduce it to them so they can use on you.

I personally get a deep tissue massage every Thursday at 9:00 a.m. I have the Zuka4 and Mobility Star that my massage therapist uses on me during my massage and I recommend you do the same. It's a GAME CHANGER. You may shed a few tears each week, but the way your body will feel is well worth the few seconds of pain.

I also recommend getting a "mansage": a massage by a MAN. The reason is because men are generally stronger and can get deeper in your tissue. If you have any issues with being touched by another man, GET over it. It's strictly business and he's there to fix you up. So get your massage!

Supplements

Although I believe in getting the majority of your nutrition from REAL food sources, there are some supplements that can help you recover quicker and help you prevent injury. One of those is glutamine. Not glucosamine – glutamine. They are quite different. Glutamine will help speed recovery from workouts, improves digestive health, improves metabolism, improves human growth hormone secretion, supports muscle growth, and improves cellular function. All of these aspects are directly tied to keeping your body in check and on point.

Although you can get glutamine from foods like turkey, wild caught salmon, cod, spirulina, grass-fed beef, and bone broth, I recommend supplementing it. Get glutamine powder only; none of the flavored kinds. Take 10-15 grams of it before and after a training session.

Sleep

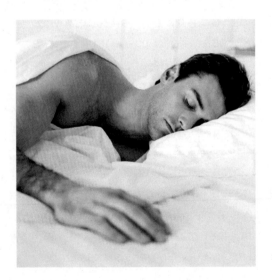

I know that as an executive/entrepreneur, getting adequate sleep is not always an easy task. But sleep is a very important element of burning fat, building muscle, recovery from training, processing information, and your health. So although I know that this one can be a tough one (I get 5.5 hours a night on average), do your best to get as much adequate sleep as possible. Squeeze in midday power naps, if possible. Get in extra naps on weekends.

I personally wake up at 4:00 a.m. seven days a week. Holidays, vacation, weekends – it doesn't matter – I get up at 4:00 a.m. But on days I feel I need more recovery, I will squeeze in power naps when possible or get an extra couple hours mid-morning on weekends. Either way, get your sleep.

The Most Painful Way to Grow muscle (EFS)

How would you like to triple your chest size within just weeks? How would you like to have bigger fuller muscles almost instantly? Well, I have a treat for you. This is something I only recently found out about through reading some scientific literature. (That's what I do on my free time: READING and learning more.) I came across this, so I decided to try it. I only did it a couple of times before one of my physique competitions and immediately noticed vast improvements in my chest from it – and I wasn't even taking it seriously yet.

After that show, I started taking it more seriously and now it is a part of my normal routine. I have been implementing it with my clients and have seen ASTOUNDING results! Some of my guys have been literally TRIPLING the size of their chest, going from flat, almost nothing, to thick, full, and well-formed chests.

When you think about gaining muscle and improving your physique, stretching is probably not one of the first things that comes to mind. But did you know that not only does stretching play a critical role in injury prevention, it also plays a critical role in building muscle? Want to know another hack that will help prevent injury and increase the size of your muscle bellies and your muscle development?

It is known as the EFS(extreme fascia stretching). Just underneath your skin lies a network of fibers, called fascia. This network of fibers wraps around every one of your muscles, bones, nerves, blood vessels, and organs. If you could imagine peeling an orange, how all the slices are completely separated into individual sections, that is our soft tissue and muscles wrapped in fascia. Fascia also connects muscle to bone via tendons, which are part of the fascia system. Basically, your fascia holds your muscles in their proper place in your body. When you are doing muscle scraping and rolling, this is primarily what you are fixing, the tight connective tissue known as fascia.

Your fascia holds you together, but it may also be holding you back from optimal muscle growth. Think about your muscles; you train them and feed them properly. They want to grow and will grow, but something is holding them back. They don't have the ROOM to grow. Fascia is very tough, so it restricts the muscles' ability to expand. It's like trying to stuff a large pillow in a small pillowcase. The size of your muscle will be limited because of the restrictions of the connective tissue around the muscles. So imagine if you can expand the size of the pillowcase by stretching it out, the pillow within has more room to grow and can fill that new space. By stretching your muscles under specific conditions, you can actually stretch your fascia and give your muscles room to grow.

The key to effective fascia stretching is implementing it when your muscles are pumped up full of blood. When your muscles are fully pumped up, they are pushing against the fascia. By stretching hard at that time, you increase the pressure on the fascia greatly and could lead to expansion of the fascia.

There is some science to this, which I will discuss in a moment. But first, I want you to imagine Arnold Schwarzenegger. Want to know why he had such an incredible chest? He used to finish his workouts with dumbbell flyes. With his chest pumped up full of blood, he would stretch at the bottom of the flye. This gave his chest room to grow to incredible proportions. He still to this day has one of the most impressive chests of ALL time and those who follow suit have very impressive chests as well.

The science, Dr. Jacob Wilson and his team put this theory to the test in the lab investigating the effects of weighted set stretching on muscle size and strength on human subjects. They took 24 recreationally trained subjects who were assigned to stretching and non-stretching conditions, training one of the most challenging body parts for most guys: the calves.

Both groups performed four sets of 12 rep calf raises on leg press twice a week for five weeks. One group stretched between sets for 30 seconds weighted, while the other group did no stretching. The results were that after five weeks, the muscle thickness DOUBLED in the group that used the stretching. Both groups noticed similar gains in strength, but the fascia stretching group led to more muscle growth.

Before one of my recent physique competitions, I read this study above in an article I came across and started to implement extreme fascia stretching into my workouts. To be honest, it wasn't even very consistently. Even though I was inconsistent with it, I still noticed increased muscle fullness, better muscle pumps, and larger looking muscles in my workouts and onstage. After seeing this firsthand and doing more research on this topic, I just recently committed to making it part of my regular training protocol. It's so awesome that I even put it in this book for you.

Here is a example of one of my 53 year-old clients who had literally almost no chest previously. We have only done this extreme fascia stretching a couple times.

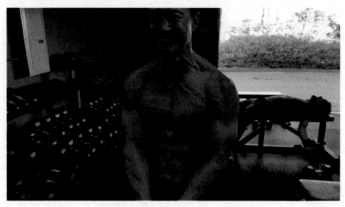

-Ivan Ho 53 years old

Look at this pump and fullness he's getting. If you look in the background, you can see another one of my new guys doing it too. Are you ready to get up to double or triple the muscle growth results from just throwing in some extreme fascia stretching towards the end of your workout when your muscles are really pumped up? Yes or yes?

How to implement

There are a few techniques to this, and it doesn't have to be difficult. The key to remember is to one, get muscles fully pumped up, which is why its best towards the end of workout. Then do a weighted or deep static stretch, this stretch should be somewhat painful and uncomfortable.

Remember, we are trying to expand the tight connective tissue surrounding your muscles. Make sure you perform this technique with exercises where you can stretch without putting yourself in a position to get injured. Make sure you don't stretch so hard that you cause the muscle to tear. You want a good firm stretch, not sharp pain. Use common sense.

Here's how it's done. At the end of a set, instead of sitting there resting or playing on your phone, do some extreme fascia stretching. Get a weight you can do about 12 times when fresh, then hold it in a stretched position for 30 seconds. Then continue to the next working set.

For example with your chest after doing a set of dumbbell bench presses, grab a pair of 20 pound dumbbells. Lay on your back and hold the dumbbells in the bottom position of a chest fly, stretching your pecs for 30 seconds. Set them down and recover. Repeat the set. Wait to implement this until after you have been training for about 30-45 minutes and muscles are pumped up, start doing this after each set and watch how awesome you start to look and feel after a few weeks.

Or you could do an actual EFS(extreme fascia stretching) round when your day is over. Weighted stretch for 30 seconds, then pump 20 reps of something to increase the blood flow to the muscles and stretch them from the inside.

Here's how you could use it for specific body parts:

Note: Keep in mind we do multiple exercises per set, so wait until the full set of two to three moves are complete before implementing the fascial stretching. Use your designated rest period to stretch. This stretch should be painful! Not painful like a sharp pain from an injury, but uncomfortably painful.

Chest: Hold a pair dumbbells in the bottom stretched position of a chest fly with a slight bend in the elbows.

Lats: Hold onto a pull-up bar and just hang for 30 seconds. Don't let your feet touch the ground. Or do a really intense Lat stretch.

Quads: With your back foot on a bench, kneel down, lean all the way back onto foot. Squeeze glute and hold for 30 seconds.

Front Delts: Similar to how you do the chest fly stretch, do the same thing. Just turn your palms towards your feet and hold.

Hamstrings: Hold the bottom position of a Romanian deadlift. Keep your hips back with your weight on the heels, with the weight close to your body.

Triceps: Put your arm behind your head, reach down your back, and lean your elbow up against the wall.

Biceps: Lay on an incline bench with dumbbells in each hand. Let the weight pull you into the stretch. You may feel your delt stretch too if you're really tight.

Calves: With weight, let your heel go as far down as possible and hold. Using either a leg press machine with heels hanging off, a calf raise machine, or just one leg at a time with a dumbbell in your hand.

Do this every workout, stretching the muscles you are training. Each week just like how we progressively overload to build, progressively increase your stretches by 3-5% in weight or add another five seconds to the stretch.

You will not only notice more flexibility, but you will start to notice more fullness, better pumps, more size, and an overall more aesthetic physique. You're going to look fuvking AWESOME!

Let's review:

1. What is the number one cause of pain and what do you need to make sure you eliminate to avoid getting injured?
2. What are the four most inflammatory foods?
3. What is rolling?
4. What is muscle scraping?
5. What tools do you need in your gym bag?
6. What is extreme fascia stretching?
7. When is the best time to implement extreme fascia stretching?

[12]

Training Phases

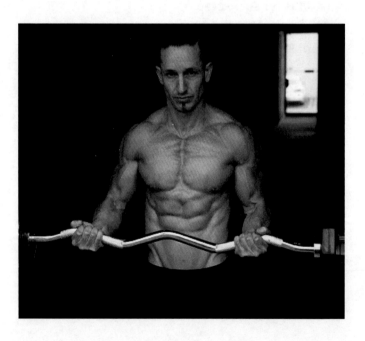

It's time to get into the training, so what should be in your gym bag? You should have a heart rate monitor (Polar FT60 or better), workout training journal, and a pen at the minimum. Being successful in business requires planning and preparation, so your physique is no different.

I want you training seven days a week. Seven days a week, you show up. I have you technically training six days, but you still show up on the seventh to at least do some flexibility and soft tissue work. Resting is optional, but rest days aren't just for laying around. You need to be productive and get your muscles in check by stretching and rolling. After you have invested some time into prepping your muscles for the next week, then you deserve some time to relax, rest, and lay around.

This is intentional. We are sending a message to your subconscious that you are dedicated, committed, serious, and will do whatever it takes. You make a habit of showing up to training seven days a week, you create a habit of showing up in life and in business every day of the week. Not only am I trying to help you get ripped, I want you wealthy and have awesome relationships. All successes in life come from establishing excellent habits and it begins with YOU in the gym.

Remember, we are heart rate training. You need to see your effort, keep heart rate above 100 BPM all day, keep track of your workout weights, reps, sets, and hit your prescribed calorie burn goal EVERY day. No excuses.

What is your calorie burn goal for each day supposed to be? What phase of training are you in and what weights are you going to lift for how many reps today?

Training Schedule.
Day 1: Legs/Abs
Day 2: Back/Chest
Day 3: Shoulders
Day 4: Legs/Calves

Day 5: Biceps/Triceps
Day 6: Shred Conditioning
Day 7: Flexibility/Mobility/Prehab

Shredded Exec Phase #1
Supersets 4x10 + HIIT 1 day.

In Phase #1, we are doing supersets for four sets of 10 reps. Supersets are two moves performed back-to-back with no rest. So for example, if we are training Day 1 Legs/Abs, you will do a Leg move, immediately to an AB move.

For instance:

SET Supersets 4x10
Set 1: Squats, 10 reps, to Hanging knee raises, 10 reps. Rest 60 seconds.
Set 2: Squats, 10 reps, to Hanging knee raises, 10 reps. Rest 60 seconds.
Set 3: Squats, 10 reps, to Hanging knee raises, 10 reps. Rest 60 seconds.
Set 4: Squats, 10 reps, to Hanging knee raises, 10 reps. Rest 60 seconds.
Done. Move to the next superset.

This is how we do Phase 1. I want you staying in Phase 1 for 30-60 days. If you have been lifting consistently for the past 5 years or more, do 30 days in this phase. If you have not, then you do 60 days. We are doing a total of six exercises PER workout, so four sets of each superset. We lift for five days and then on the sixth day, we do a conditioning day doing sprints and other forms of HIIT training. Pay close attention to your heart rate and your rest times.

What are you supposed to keep your heart rate above while lifting? Right! 100 BPM.

When doing Conditioning/HIIT what is the Goal heart rate you should be peaking over? Right! 180 BPM.

What is the rule about your calorie burn? Right! You must hit your calorie burn goal of 500-1,000+ EVERY training day.

Once you have completed 30-60 days in SET Phase 1, you move on to Phase 2.

Shredded Exec Training Phase #2
Tri-sets 4x8 + HIIT one day

In Shredded Exec Phase #2, we are increasing the weights, lowering the reps, then adding a third move to the end of each set. We are still doing the HEAVY supersets for the first two moves, then a lighter weight/plyometric move at the end. We are adding this third move to reduce rest time and create an ACTIVE recovery environment so we BURN more calories. When we burn more calories, what happens? We burn more FAT! Yes or yes?

So we are still doing the primary superset, but followed by a third move that will keep our heart rate elevated. This third move will be LIGHTER; we are only utilizing this move to burn more calories, so it's not intended as a heavy weight exercise. Remember when I told you light weights had their place? This is what I meant.

You'll also notice your rest has been reduced, because your third move is an active recovery move. Your primary muscles are recovering while we are training the third move. You will see the difference when you look at your calorie burn and average and maximum heart rates at the end of your workout. Expect a higher calorie burn for the day. So if you normally burn 700, you may hit 800-1000+ with this tri-set training.

Typically for this third move, it will be one that we trained the day prior. This is to give it a pump as well, to deliver nutrients so it recovers faster. For example, if you did legs on Monday, Tuesday you would be doing a tri-set of chest and back heavy, then the third move would be a lighter leg move to keep heart rate up and get a pump to speed recovery of the legs. Does that make sense? Awesome!

Don't worry, I did all the work for you in designing the workouts. All you have to do is DTFW!

For Instance:

Tri-set #1: Squats 8 reps, to Hanging knee Raises 8 reps, Barbell Rows 20 reps. Rest 30 seconds.
Tri-set #2: Squats 8 reps, to Hanging knee Raises 8 reps, Barbell Rows 20 reps. Rest 30 seconds.
Tri-set #3: Squats 8 reps, to Hanging knee Raises 8 reps, Barbell Rows 20 reps. Rest 30 seconds.
Tri-set #4: Squats 8 reps, to Hanging knee Raises 8 reps, Barbell Rows 20 reps. Rest 30 seconds.
Done. Move to the next Tri-Set.

You will notice you may be sucking more wind. You will notice you are going to be burning MORE calories, FASTER. Stay in SET Phase 2 for 30 days if you have five or more years of consistent lifting experience, 60 days if you do not.

Shredded Exec Training Phase #3

Extreme Stimulation Training - SD20 for 4 sets

By this point, you should have 60-120 days of consistent training under your belt. You should be looking good, feeling good, strong, lean, and training like a beast. Now we are progressing to the Super Drop-Sets for 20 reps, a/k/a SD20. In this phase, we are going back to just two moves, BUT you'll end up doing six mini sets with these two moves for every set. This training is INTENSE!

To do SD20, start off with your three rep max weight and do three reps. Immediately reduce the weight, then do seven reps. Immediately reduce the weight again, then do 10 reps. That's a total of 20 reps. Now do the same exact thing for the other move paired with this one. Three reps, seven reps, then 10 reps. That's ONE full set. Rest 90 seconds, then do four sets. OMG! This method is very intense, so you may need to find a trashcan.

For Instance:

SD20 EST Set #1
DB Bench Press: 120x3, 90x7, 60x10
DB Single Arm Row: 120x3, 90x7, 60x10, left side.
Then do the right side.
Rest 90 seconds.

SD20 EST Set #2
DB Bench Press: 120x3, 90x7, 60x10
DB Single Arm Row: 120x3, 90x7, 60x10, left side.
Then do the right side.
Rest 90 seconds.

SD20 EST Set #3

DB Bench Press: 120x3, 90x7, 60x10

DB Single Arm Row: 120x3, 90x7, 60x10, left side.

Then do the right side.

Rest 90 seconds.

SD20 EST Set #4

DB Bench Press: 120x3, 90x7, 60x10

DB Single Arm Row: 120x3, 90x7, 60x10, left side.

Then do the right side.

Rest 90 seconds

Done!

Now move to the next SD20 round. This method is madness, insane, and fun. Just make sure you have followed the plan and worked your way up to this. You'll notice your rest periods increased a little bit because you will need it. This type of training MELTS calories, MELTS fat, and is a lot of fun to do. Stay in this phase until you are shredded.

Accelerate fat loss with doubles

Now I know some of you may be impatient, physiques take time to develop, but there is a method to accelerate your fat loss so you can get shredded FASTER. I ONLY recommend this for very fit, advanced level people.

What makes the body burn fat? Deficit! So HOW could we create MORE of a deficit? Reduce calories?

NO! Keep your calories where they belong and increase your OUTPUT! Doubles are how you achieve this. Basically, this means doing ANOTHER workout, doubling up your training for the day. Let's say you are doing your S.E.T at 5:00 a.m. so, later on in the evening you would do a double and do some conditioning work or another SET workout. You would be doubling your workouts each day.

It can be as simple as just lacing up, walking outside, and doing 20 x 50 yard sprints in front of your house, or you could go back and hit the gym and train the same body parts you trained at 5:00 a.m. again. Or you could just do a different type of HIIT workout.

Either way, the most important element is that you are expending calories, so what you do doesn't matter much, just BURNING more calories. Just make sure that it is NOT steady state cardio or any form of endurance training, such as running distances, biking, etc.

Either lift sprint! You can also do a form of HIIT (sleds, ropes, plyos, or other forms of high intensity intervals).

You may only want to start doing doubles three times a week at first. I would also keep them short and intense. Like I said, this is only recommended for very fit, advanced level people. Just doing the SET Phases 1-3 is enough to get you shredded at a very good pace, but I know some of you are impatient, so this is your option.

Make sure you invest a lot of time on your prehab, rolling, stretching, scraping, and massaging to keep your body in check. Do whatever it takes to get your body shredded. Once you are there, then we move to the SET Phase 4: Growth.

SET Phase 4 Build 5x5

Chances are that once you get shredded, you are more than likely going to want to increase muscle in a few areas or all of your body. There is always room for improvement, and always things we can make better. You may want bigger arms, chest, legs, calves, back, and shoulders or just want to increase your weight. If you are content with how your physique is, just move back to Phase 1 and continue lifting heavy for four sets of 5-10 reps to maintain.

I have yet to meet someone who is content and have found that most men always have areas they can and want to improve. That's what Phase 4 is for. This is the fun one. This is the one that you get to reduce your intensity and just focus on progressively overloading your muscles and lifting heavy at a slower pace to focus on just adding size.

In this phase we are going REALLY heavy with five sets of five reps. Pick your five rep max weight, then do five sets of five reps with it. Each week, you should try to push out one or two more reps per set. Once you can do all five sets for eight reps or more with that weight, it's time to INCREASE weights.

For instance, if you are doing DB Bench Press for 100 x 5,5,5,5,5 this week. Next week, your goal is 100 x 6,6,6,6,6. You may only get six on the first set or the first few, but the goal is to progressively overload your muscles week after week. This is what forces the body to keep progressing, to develop more strength, and to develop more muscle.

Want more strength? Want more muscle? Then what should you be doing every workout so you know exactly what you did last time and what you need to do today? Right! Journaling! This is WHY it is so crucial that you track your training. You have a record of what you did last time, so you have a GOAL to beat this time. This is how you make GAINS.

In this phase, once you are shredded, we reverse diet SLOWLY. Now during this phase, you're not only going to increase your weights and sets, but you are going to also slowly increase your calories. We are going to do what is called reverse dieting, which is essentially just you slowly increasing your calories over time.

How to reverse diet

When it comes to adding more muscle, we DO NOT BULK. This term "bulk" is a term used by weak-minded men that try to justify eating trash and getting fat. This is usually a term used by guys who eat terrible, have no self-discipline, high body fat, and usually have NEVER seen their abs. This is the DUMB way of adding size. What's the point of adding size if 50-80% of it is fat and you can't see the muscle anyway?

In my opinion, what's the point of gaining muscle if you're too fat to see them and you look like shit with your shirt off. Men should be RIPPED and have visible abs YEAR-ROUND, NO EXCUSES.

"If you don't have abs, you're fat. Period!"
–Daymond Sewall

So if you or someone you know has been using the "I'm bulking" term but you don't have visible abs, you're not bulking – you're FAT. Get shredded first, then start adding size like I'm about to show you. We do this the INTELLIGENT and strategic way. Want to know the smart way?

The amount of calories your body is ACTUALLY going to use to build muscle is very small. So when it comes to adding calories into your diet, you can only add a couple hundred calories at a time, which is why bulking is stupid. Most these idiots add thousands of calories to their diet. The human body does not need that much to repair and grow muscle. This is why the bulking calories are often stored as fat.

To do this intelligently, we start off increasing your calories slowly. We do this to KEEP your shreds and build over time. So we start by adding in another 100-200 calories per day, just increase your carbs by a little to get an extra 100-200 calories into your diet. Then keep training, watch your physique, stay at this intake for three weeks, reassess and if you're still looking awesome, bump it up another 100-200 calories. Stay there for three weeks and reassess.

Keep doing this until you hit an amount that makes it seem like you may add some body fat if you go any higher or if you notice your body fat increases a little. For smaller guys, this top number is around 2,700. For taller or more muscular guys, this may be as high as 5,000.

The key is to slowly increase your calories over time to KEEP your shreds while adding size. You get to fill out and develop more muscle, all while staying shredded. Just like throughout this entire book, there is science, methods, and strategies on how to do EVERYTHING. However, you are NOT allowed to move to this phase of training until you are shredded.

SET Training Program Phases 1-4
Training Schedule
Day 1: Legs/Abs
Day 2: Back/Chest
Day 3: Shoulders
Day 4: Legs/Calves
Day 5: Biceps/Triceps
Day 6: Shred Conditioning
Day 7: Flexibility/Mobility/Prehab

Shredded Exec Training Phase #1
Supersets 4x10 + HIIT 1 day

In Phase 1, we are doing supersets for four sets of 10 reps. Supersets are two moves performed back-to-back with no rest. So for example, if we are training Day 1 Legs/Abs, you will do a leg move, immediately to an AB move, and then rest 60 seconds.

For instance:

SET Super-Sets 4x10

Set 1: Squats 10 reps, to Hanging Knee Raises 10 reps. Rest 60 seconds.
Set 2: Squats 10 reps, to Hanging Knee Raises 10 reps. Rest 60 seconds.
Set 3: Squats 10 reps, to Hanging Knee Raises 10 reps. Rest 60 seconds.
Set 4: Squats 10 reps, to Hanging Knee Raises 10 reps. Rest 60 seconds.
Done. Move to the next Super-Set.

I want you staying in Phase 1 for 30-60 days. If you have been lifting consistently for the past five years or more, do 30 days in this phase. If you have not, then you do 60 days. We are doing a total of six exercises PER workout, with 4 sets of each superset. Lift for five days, then on the sixth day we do a conditioning day, doing sprints and other forms of HIIT training. Pay close attention to your heart rate and your rest times.

What are you supposed to keep your heart rate above while Lifting? Right! 100 BPM.

When doing conditioning/HIIT, what is the goal heart rate you should be peaking over? Right! 180 BPM. What is the rule about your calorie burn? Right! You must hit your calorie burn goal EVERY training day of 500-1,000+ calories.

Okay, it sounds like you are ready. Let's get to it! Get your notebook and write down these workouts so you can keep track of your sets, reps, and weights.

If you do not know what an exercise is, what should you do to find out? GOOGLE! YOUTUBE!

Shredded Exec Training Phase 1
Supersets 4x10

Training Day #1: Leg and Abs
Warm-up 100 steps Walking Lunges
Set #1. 4 x 10 reps
Warm-up 20 reps Squats
A1. Squats, 10 reps
A2. Plank Arm Reach, 10 reps each side
Rest 60 seconds.

Set #2. 4 x 10 reps
Warm-up 20 reps Leg Press.
B1. Leg Press 10 reps.
B2. Decline Sit-up with DB under chin 10 reps
Rest 60 seconds.

Set #3 4 X 10 reps
Warm-up 20 reps BB Lunges
C1. Barbell Reverse Lunges, 10 reps each side
C2. Reverse Crunches ,10 reps
Rest 60 seconds.

Set #4 100 Reps Drop Set

D1. Machine Calf Raises with 10 rep max weight, go until drop weight, go until failure, repeat until you have done one hellish set of calves. Now stretch quads, hamstrings, and calves. Do soft tissue work if needed.

Training Day #2 Chest and Back

Warm-up. 25 Pushups, 25 Wide Lat Pulldowns, 3 sets

Set #1. 4 x 10 reps

Warm-up. 20 BB Incline Bench, 20 BB Row

A1. Barbell Incline Bench Press 10 reps

A2. Barbell Row 10 reps

Rest 60 seconds.

Set #2. 4 x 10 reps

Warm-up BB Flat Bench, 20 reps, rows, 20 reps.

B1. Barbell Flat Bench, 10 reps

B2. Two Arm DB Row, 10 reps (same time)

Rest 60 seconds.

Set #3 4 X 10 REPS.

Warm-up. 20 reps DB Flye, 20 Wide Lat Pulldown

C1. Dumbbell Flye Flat Bench, 10 reps.

C2. Wide Lat Pulldown, 10 reps.

Rest 60 seconds.

Stretch chest and lats

Training Day #3 Shoulders

Warm-up 25 DB Shoulder Press, 3 sets

Set #1. 4 x 10 reps.

Warm-up 20 BB Shoulder Press, 20 Bent Rear Delt Flyes

A1. Barbell Shoulder Press, 10 reps
A2. Bent Over Rear Delt Flye, 10 reps
Rest 60 seconds.

Set #2. 4 x 10 reps
Warm-up 20 Side Raises DB, 20 Incline Rear Delt Flye
B1. Dumbbell Side Raises (lateral raises), 10 reps
B2. Incline Rear Delt, 10 reps. (face down on inc. bench)
Rest 60 seconds.

Set #3 4 X 10 REPS.
Warm-up
C1. Barbell Front Raise (eye level)
C2. Single Arm Cable Rear Delt flye, 10 each
Rest 60 seconds.

Training Day #4 Legs Day 2.
Warm-up 100 steps Walking Lunges

Set #1. 4 x 10 reps.
Warm-up 20 reps Deadlifts
A1. Deadlifts, 10 reps (Go light until form is on point. Roll hip flexors, quads, and hamstrings prior)
A2. Standing Calf Machine, 10 reps
Rest 60 seconds.

Set #2. 4 x 10 reps
Warm-up 20 reps DB squats
B1. DB squats, 10 reps (Holding 2 DB at sides)
B2. Sitting calf (soleus), 10 reps SLOW
Rest 60 seconds.

Set #3 4 x 10 reps
Warm-up 20 reps DB Lunges
C1. DB Reverse Lunges, 10 reps each side
C2. DB Single Leg Standing Calf Raise, 10 reps each side
Rest 60 seconds.
Stretch quads, hamstrings, calves and roll muscles.

Training Day #5 Arms

Warm-up. 25 Tricep Pressdowns, 25 DB Bicep Curls, 3 sets

Set #1. 4 x 10 reps.
Warm-up BB Curls, 20 reps and BB Skull Crusher, 20 reps
A1. BB Bicep Curls, 10 reps, EZ Curl Bar
A2. BB Skull Crusher ,10 reps, EZ Curl Bar
Rest 60 seconds.

Set #2. 4 x 10 reps
Warm-up Tricep Pressdown Bar 20,
DB bicep curls,palms up, 20 reps
B1. Tricep Pressdown on the cable with bar attach, 10 reps
B2. DB Bicep Curls Palms up, both same time, 10 reps
Rest 60 seconds.

Set #3 4 X 10 REPS.
Warm-up 20 Cable Curls with bar,
20 skull crushers DB
C1. Cable Curls with bar, 10 reps
C2. Skull Crusher with DB, 10 reps
Rest 60 seconds.
Stretch biceps and triceps.

Training Day #6 Shred Conditioning.

Preferably outdoor local football field/track.

Indoor option below if weather doesn't permit.

Warm-up 100 steps Walking Lunges, 50 Lunge Jumps,

3 x 50 yard sprints at 50-70% max speed

10 x 50 yard Sprints, walk back

5 x 100 yard Sprints, walk back

5 x 100 yard Burpees with a Burpee every 10 yards

Rest 60 seconds between sets.

Training Day #7
Prehab, mobility, and flexibility

1. Roll quads individually from knee to hip 20 times. Knee to hip and back to knee is only 1 rep. 20 reps, both sides.
2. Stretch both quads, 2 sets of 30 seconds, each side.
3. Roll hip flexors. The best way is to lay a DB down so it rolls, using the edge of a 10-20 lb. dumbbell, lay on it placing the dumbbell edge just inside your hip bone. Break up the knots.
4. Stretch hip flexor, 2 sets 30 seconds.
5. Roll IT bands, 20 passes knee to hip.
6. Roll lats, 20 passes from very top, down to low back.
7. Stretch lats, 2 sets of 30 seconds.
8. Roll pecs. Lay on top of a 5-15 lb. dumbbell right on your chest. Keep arms out wide, making gym angels. This is going to hurt, so suck it up. It will make your

chest bigger and fuller looking from the increased range of motion, shoulder width, and blood flow.

9. Stretch pecs doing the doorway stretch on a pole or wall 2 sets 30 seconds.
10. Roll calves on roller or handle of a 5-15 lb. dumbbell for 20 passes.
11. Stretch calves, 2 sets 30 seconds.

Now you're all set and ready to kill it in training next week. Awesome job!!!

Shredded Exec Training Phase 2
Tri-sets 4x8

In Shredded Exec Phase 2, we are increasing the weights, lowering the reps, then adding a third move to the end of each set. We are still doing the HEAVY supersets for the first two moves, then a lighter weight/plyometric move at the end. We are adding this third move to reduce rest time and create an ACTIVE rest environment so we BURN more calories.

You'll also notice your rest has been reduced, this is because your third move is an active recovery move. Your primary muscles are recovering while we are training the third move. You will see the difference when you look at your calorie burn and average and maximum heart rate on your HRM at the end of your workout. Expect a higher calorie burn for the day. So if you normally burn 700, you may hit 800-1000+ with this tri-set training.

For Instance:

Tri-Set #1. Squats 8 reps, to hanging knee raises 8 reps, barbell rows, 20 reps.

Rest 30 seconds.

Tri-Set #2. Squats 8 reps, to hanging knee raises 8 reps, barbell rows, 20 reps.

Rest 30 seconds.

Tri-Set #3. Squats 8 reps, to hanging knee raises 8 reps, barbell rows, 20 reps.

Rest 30 seconds.

Tri-Set #4. Squats 8 reps, to hanging knee raises 8 reps, barbell rows, 20 reps.

Rest 30 seconds.

Done. Move to the next tri-set.

Shredded Exec Training Phase #2
Tri-Sets 4x8

Training Day 1 Leg and Abs.

Warm-up 100 steps Walking Lunges

Set #1. 4 x 8 reps
Warm-up 20 reps Squats
A1. Squats, 8 reps
A2. DB Romanian Deadlifts, 8 reps
A3. Hanging Knee Raises, 20 reps
Rest 30 seconds.

Set #2. 4 x 8 reps
Warm-up 20 reps Leg Press
B1. Leg Press Shoulder Width, 8 reps
B2. Barbell Romanian Deadlifts, 8 reps
B3. Decline Sit-up with DB under chin, 20 reps
Rest 30 seconds.

Set #3 4 x 8 REPS.
Warm-up 20 reps BB Lunges
C1. Barbell Reverse Lunges, 8 reps each side
C2. Laying Hamstring Curls, 8 reps
C3. Reverse Crunches, 20 reps
Rest 30 seconds.

Set #4 100 Reps Drop Set
D1. Machine calf raises with 5 rep max weight, go until failure, drop weight, go until failure, repeat until you have done one hellish set of calves.

Now stretch quads, hamstrings, and calves.
Do soft tissue work if needed.

Training Day #2 Chest and Back
Warm-up 25 Pushups, 25 Wide Lat Pulldowns, 3 sets

Set #1. 4 x 8 reps.

Warm-up. 20 DB incline bench, 20 DB row
A1. Dumbbell Incline Bench Press, 8 reps
A2. Dumbbell Single Arm Row, 8 reps each
A3. Walking Lunges Bodyweight, 20 steps
Rest 30 seconds.

Set #2. 4 x 8 reps
Warm-up. DB Flat Bench 20 reps, BB Rows, 20 reps
B1. DB Flat Bench, 8 reps
B2. BB Row 8 reps
B3. DB Squats, 20 reps, light
Rest 30 seconds.

Set #3 4 x 8 REPS.
Warm-up 20 reps Cable Chest Flye, 20 Wide Lat Pulldown
C1. Cable Flye 8 reps
C2. Pull-ups wide, 8 reps. Use machine if you have to.
C3. DB Reverse Lunges, 20 steps total
Rest 30 seconds.
Stretch chest and lats.

Training Day #3 Shoulders
Warm-up 25 Side Raises, 3 sets

Set #1. 4 x 8 reps.
Warm-up 20 DB Shoulder Press, 20 Bent Rear Delt Flyes
A1. Dumbbell Shoulder Press, 8 reps
A2. Bent Over Rear Delt Flye, 8 reps
A3. Dumbbell Bent Over Row, 20 reps
Rest 30 seconds.

Set #2. 4 x 8 reps
Warmup. 20 Barbell Shoulder Presses,
20 Incline Rear Delt Flyes
B1. BB Shoulder Press, 8 reps
B2. Incline Rear Delt, 8 reps
(lying face down on an incline bench)
B3. Cable Row V-grip, 20 reps.
Rest 30 seconds.

Set #3 4 X 8 REPS.
Warm-up DB Side Raises 20 reps
C1. DB Side Raises
C2. Single Arm Cable Rear Delt Flye, 8 each

C3. Pushups, 20 reps
Rest 30 seconds.

Training Day #4 Legs Day 2.
Warm-up 100 steps Walking Lunges

Set #1. 4 x 8 reps
Warm-up 20 reps Sumo Deadlifts
A1. Sumo Deadlifts, 8 reps (roll hip flexors, quads, and hamstrings prior)
A2. Standing Calf Machine, 8 reps
A3. DB Shoulder Press, 20 reps
Rest 30 seconds.

Set #2. 4 x 8 reps
Warm-up 20 reps DB Squats
B1. BB Walking Lunges, 8 each side, knee touching the floor
B2. Sitting Calf (Soleus), 8 reps SLOW
B3. BB Shoulder Presses, 20 reps
Rest 30 seconds.

Set #3 4 X 8 reps
Warm-up 20 reps Leg Curls
C1. Laying Hamstring Curls, 8 reps
C2. DB Single Leg Standing Calf Raise, 8 each side
C3. Side Raises, 20 reps
Rest 30 seconds.
Stretch quads, hamstrings, and calves. Roll muscles.

Training Day #5 Arms
Warm-up 25 Tricep Pressdowns, 25 DB Bicep Curls, 3 sets

Set #1. 4 x 8 reps

Warm-up DB Curls, 20 reps DB Skull Crusher, 20 reps

A1. DB Bicep Curls, 8 reps, same time

A2. DB Skull Crusher, 8 reps, same time

A3. Squat Jumps, 20 reps

Rest 30 seconds.

Set #2. 4 x 8 reps

Warm-up Tricep Pressdown Rope,

20 reps BB Bicep Curls, 20 reps

B1. Tricep Pressdown Rope, 8 reps

B2. BB Bicep Curls, 8 reps

B3. Lunge Jumps, 20 reps

Rest 30 seconds.

Set #3 4 x 8 reps

Warm-up 20 Cable Pressdown with bar,

20 Hammer Curls DB

C1. Cable Pressdown with bar, 8 reps

C2. Hammer Curls with DB, 8 reps

C3. Box Jumps, 20 reps

Rest 30 seconds.

Training Day #6 Shred Conditioning

Preferably outdoor local football field/track.

Indoor option below if weather doesn't permit.

Warm-up 100 steps walking lunges, 50 lunge jumps,

3 x 50 yard Sprints 50-70% max speed

10 x 100 yard Sprints, walk back

10 x 50 yard Sprints, walk back

25 Stadiums. (It only counts on the up, so sprint up, come down; that's 1 rep.)

Find a trashcan.☺

Stretch quads, hamstrings, and calves.

Training Day #7
Prehab, mobility, flexibility

1. Roll quads individually from knee to hip 20x. Knee to hip, and back to knee is only 1 rep. 20 reps both sides.
2. Stretch both quads, 2 sets of 30 seconds each side.
3. Roll hip flexors. The best way is to lay a DB down so it rolls, using the edge of a 10-20 lb. dumbbell, lay on it placing the dumbbell edge just inside your hip bone. Break up the knots.
4. Stretch hip flexors, 2 sets 30 seconds.
5. Roll IT bands, 20 passes knee to hip.
6. Roll lats, 20 passes from very top, down to low back.
7. Stretch lats, 2 sets of 30 seconds.
8. Roll pecs. Lay on top of a 5-15 lb. dumbbell right on chest. Keep arms out wide, make gym angels. This is going to hurt, so suck it up. It will make your chest bigger and fuller, looking from the increased range of motion, shoulder width and blood flow.
9. Stretch pecs doing the doorway stretch on a pole or wall, 2 sets 30 seconds.
10. Roll calves on roller or handle of a 5-15 lb. dumbbell, 20 passes.
11. Stretch calves, 2 sets 30 seconds.

Now you're all set and ready to kill it in training next week. Awesome job!!!

Shredded Exec Training Phase #3
Extreme Stimulation Training
Shred Style SD20 Method (Super Drop-sets, 20 reps)

By this point, you should have 60-120 days of consistent training under your belt. You should be looking good, feeling good, strong, lean, and training like a beast. Now we are progressing to the super drop-sets for 20 reps, a/k/a my favorite method of SD20. In this phase, we are going back to just two moves, BUT you'll end up doing six mini sets with these two moves every set. This training is INTENSE!

To do SD20, Start off with your three rep max weight, do three reps. Immediately reduce the weight, then do seven reps. Immediately reduce the weight again, then do 10 reps. That's a total of 20 reps. Now do the same exact thing for the other move paired with this one. Three reps, 7 reps, then 10 reps. That's ONE full set. Do four sets. OMG! You may need to find a trashcan.

For Instance:

SD20 EST Set #1
A1. DB Bench Press 120x3, 90x7, 60x10
A2. DB Single Arm Row 120x3, 90x7, 60x10, left side,
 then right
Rest 60 seconds.
4 Sets

Shredded Exec Training Day 1
Leg and Abs
SD20 Method (3 Reps, 7 reps, 10 reps)

Warm-up. 100 steps Walking Lunges

Set #1. 4 x SD20 reps
Warm-up 20 reps Squats
A1. Squats SD20 reps
(use 10s, 25s to load bar for easy stripping.)
A2. Decline Sit-up DB SD20
(heavy DB, medium DB, bodyweight)
Rest 90 seconds.

Set #2. 4 x SD20 reps
Warm-up 20 reps Leg Press
B1. Leg Press shoulder-width SD20 (load up with 45s)
B2. Hanging Leg Raises SD20
Rest 90 seconds.

Set #3 4 X SD20
Warm-up 20 reps BB Lunges
C1. Barbell Walking Lunges SD20
(6 Steps, 14 steps, 20 steps,
so it is each leg)
C2. Cable Crunches SD20, kneeling

Rest 90 seconds.
Stretch quads, hamstrings and calves.

Training Day #2 Chest and Back
SD20 Method
Warm-up 25 Push-ups, 25 Wide Lat Pulldowns, 3 sets

Set #1. 4 x SD20
Warm-up 20 DB Incline Bench, 20 DB Row
A1. DB Incline Bench Press SD20 reps
(Rack after each so you're not hogging 6 DBs.)
A2. Weighted Pull-ups
(Do bodyweight all 20 if you have to and
rest as needed.)
Rest 90 seconds.

Set #2. 4 x SD20
Warm-up. DB Flat Bench 20 reps, Rows 20 reps
B1. DB Flat Bench SD20
B2. DB Single Arm Row SD20
(Left 3, right 3, left 7, right 7, left 10, right 10)
Rest 90.

Set #3. 4 x SD20
Warm-up. 20 reps Cable Flye, 20 DB Rows
C1. Cable fly SD20
C2. Two-arm DB Row SD20 (same time)
Rest 90 seconds.
Stretch chest and lats.

Training Day #3 Shoulders

SD20 Method
Warm-up. 25 BB Shoulder Press, 3 sets

Set #1. 4 x SD20
Warm-up 20 DB Shoulder Press, 20 Bent Rear Delt Flyes
A1. DB Shoulder Press SD20
A2. Bent Over Rear Delt Flye SD20
Rest 90 seconds.

Set #2. 4 x SD20
Warm-up 20 Side Raises DB, 20 Incline Rear Delt Flye
B1. Barbell Shoulder Press SD20
B2. Incline Rear Delt SD20
Rest 90 seconds.

Set #3 4 x SD20
Warm-up
C1. DB Side Raises SD20
C2. Face Pull SD20
Rest 90 seconds.

Training Day #4 Legs Day 2
SD20 Method
Warm-up. 100 Goblet squats DB

Set #1. 4 x SD20
Warm-up 20 reps Deadlifts
A1. Sumo Deadlifts SD20
(Be safe; roll prior to doing this exercise.)
A2. Standing Calf Machine SD20
Rest 90 seconds.

Set #2. 4 x SD20

Warm-up 20 reps DB Squats

B1. DB Split Squats SD20

(3 left, 3 right, drop weight, 7, 7, 10, 10)

B2. Sitting Calf (Soleus) SD20

Rest 90 seconds.

Set #3 4 x SD20

Warm-up 20 reps DB Lunges

C1. DB Walking Lunges SD20 (6, 14, 20 steps)

C2. DB Single Leg Standing Calf Raises

SD20 (3,3,7,7,10,10)

Rest 90 seconds.

Stretch quads, hamstrings, and calves. Roll muscles.

Training Day #5 Arms

SD20 Method

Warm-up. 25 Close Grip Pushups,

25 DB Bicep Curls, 3 sets

Set #1. 4 x SD20

Warm-up BB Curls, 20 reps.

DB Skull Crusher, 20 reps

A1. BB Bicep Curls SD20

A2. DB Skull Crusher SD20

Rest 90 seconds.

Set #2. 4 x SD20

Warm-up BB Skull Crusher, 20 reps,

DB Bicep Curls, palms up, 20 reps

B1. BB Skull Crusher SD20

B2. DB Bicep Curls Palms up, both same time SD20

Rest 90 seconds.

Set #3 4 x SD20

Warm-up 20 Cable Curls with bar,
20 DB Triceps Ext behind head
C1. Cable Curls with Rope SD20
C2. Triceps Ext behind head with 1 heavy DB SD20
Rest 90 seconds.
Stretch biceps and triceps.

Training Day #6 Shred Conditioning

Preferably outdoor local football field/track.
Indoor option below if weather doesn't permit.
Warm-up 100 steps Walking Lunges, 50 Lunge Jumps,
3 x 50 yard Sprints 50-70% max speed
10 x 50 yard Sprints, jog back
25 Stadiums
10 x 100 yard Sprints, jog back
25 Stadiums
Find a trashcan.☺
Stretch quads, hamstrings, and calves.

Training Day #7
Prehab, mobility, flexibility.

1. Roll quads individually from knee to hip 20x. Knee to hip and back to knee is only 1 rep. 20 reps both sides.
2. Stretch both quads, 2 sets of 30 seconds each side.
3. Roll hip flexors. The best way is to lay a DB down so it rolls, using the edge of a 10-20 lb. dumbbell, lay on it

placing the dumbbell edge just inside your hip bone. Break up the knots.

4. Stretch hip flexors, 2 sets 30 seconds.
5. Roll IT bands, 20 passes knee to hip.
6. Roll lats, 20 passes from very top, down to low back.
7. Stretch lats, 2 sets of 30 seconds.
8. Roll pecs. Lay on top of a 5-15 lb. dumbbell right on chest. Keep arms out wide, make gym angels. This is going to hurt, so suck it up. It will make your chest bigger and fuller, looking from the increased range of motion, shoulder width, and blood flow.
9. Stretch pecs doing the doorway stretch on a pole or wall, 2 sets 30 seconds.
10. Roll calves on roller, or handle of a 5-15 lb. dumbbell, 20 passes.
11. Stretch calves, 2 sets 30 seconds.

Now you're all set and ready to kill it in training next week. Awesome job!

Phase #4 Shredded Executive Swole Program
SET Phase 4 Build 5x5

This phase is only for you AFTER you get shredded. This is the fun one. This is the one that you get to reduce your intensity and just focus on progressively overloading your muscles, lifting heavy, slower pace to focus on just adding size. In this phase, we aren't trying to keep your heart rate up and we aren't focusing on burning calories. This phase is all about GAINS. This phase is all about adding some muscle to your frame.

In this phase, we are going REALLY heavy, with five sets of five reps. Pick your five rep max weight, then do five sets of five reps with it. You get two minutes of rest after each set to fully recover and the focus is continual progressive overload. Each week, you should try to push out one or two more reps per set. Once you can do all five sets for eight reps or more with that weight, it's time to INCREASE weights.

Feel free to change up the exercises to hit areas you want to bring up. Use the exercise list I gave you earlier in this book for alternatives. Anything you don't know, Google does, so google it or YouTube it. So if you want to focus more on say upper pecs, do only INCLINE chest movements. If you want more width in your lats, do more wide grip pulldowns, pull-ups, etc. Just make sure you do six exercises for 30 total sets each day.

You will also be reverse dieting, so do this slowly and very carefully, because your calorie output is going to be lower due to the decreased intensity and increased rest periods. I would also recommend utilizing this rest period for extreme fascia stretching to accelerate your growth.

You can also just stay in Phase 3 of the program and build as well; just take longer rests after each SD20 set. Like I have told you many times, there are many ways of doing this, so the key is just progression and consistency. I've given you the best information and strategies that has ever existed and it's now up to you to make it your lifestyle.

How to do the 5x5

For instance, if you are doing DB bench press 100 x 5,5,5,5,5 this week, so next week your goal is 100 x 6,6,6,6,6. You may only get six on the first set or the first few, but the goal is to progressively overload your muscles week after week. This is what forces the body to keep progressing, to develop more strength, and to develop more muscle.

Day 1 Leg and Abs

5 x 5 Heavy
Warm-up 100 steps Walking Lunges

Set #1. 5 x 5 reps
Warm-up 20 reps Squats
A1. Squats
A2. Decline Sit-up DB
Rest 120 seconds.

Set #2. 5x5 reps
Warm-up 20 reps Leg Press
B1. Leg Press, shoulder width
B2. Hanging Leg Raises
Rest 120 seconds.

Set #3. 5 x 5 reps
Warm-up 20 reps BB Lunges
C1. Barbell Walking Lunges, 10 steps
C2. Cable Crunches, heavy, 5 reps, kneeling
Rest 120 seconds.
Stretch quads, hamstrings, and calves.

Training Day #2 Chest and Back

Warm-up. 25 Push-ups, 25 Wide Lat Pulldowns, 3 sets

Set #1. 5 x 5
Warm-up 20 DB Incline Bench, 20 DB Row
A1. DB Incline Bench Press
A2. Weighted Pull-ups

Rest 120 seconds.

Set #2. 5 x 5
Warm-up DB Flat Bench 20 reps, Rows, 20 reps
B1. DB Flat Bench
B2. DB Single Arm Row
Rest 120 seconds.

Set #3. 5 x 5
Warm-up 20 reps Cable Flye, 20 DB rows
C1. Cable Flye
C2. Two-arm DB Row (same time)
Rest 120 seconds.
Stretch chest and lats.

Training Day #3 Shoulders
SD20 Method
Warm-up. 25 BB Shoulder Press, 3 sets

Set #1. 5 x 5
Warm-up 20 DB Shoulder Press, 20 Bent Rear Delt Flyes
A1. DB Shoulder Press
A2. Bent Over Rear Delt Flye
Rest 120 seconds.

Set #2. 5 x 5
Warm-up. 20 Side Raises DB, 20 Incline Rear Delt Flye
B1. Barbell Shoulder Press
B2. Incline Rear Delt
Rest 120 seconds.

Set #3. 5 x 5

Warm-up
C1. DB Side Raises
C2. Face Pull
Rest 120 seconds.

Training Day #4 Legs Day 2

5 x 5 reps
Warm-up 100 Goblet Squats DB

Set #1. 5 x 5
Warm-up 20 reps Deadlifts
A1. Sumo Deadlifts (Be safe; roll prior to doing this exercise.)
A2. Standing Calf Machine SD20
Rest 120 seconds.

Set #2. 5 x 5
Warm-up 20 reps DB Squats
B1. DB Split Squats
B2. Sitting Calf (Soleus)
Rest 120 seconds.

Set #3. 5 x 5
Warm-up 20 reps DB Lunges
C1. DB Walking Lunges, 10 steps
C2. DB Single Leg Standing Calf Raises
Rest 120 seconds.
Stretch quads, hamstrings, and calves. Roll muscles.

Training Day #5 Arms 5 x 5

Warm-up 25 Close-grip Push-ups,
25 DB Bicep Curls, 3 sets

Set #1. 5 x 5
Warm-up BB Curls 20 reps. DB Skull Crusher, 20 reps
A1. BB Bicep Curls
A2. DB Skull Crusher
Rest 120 seconds.

Set #2. 5 x 5
Warm-up BB Skull Crusher 20,
DB Bicep Curls, palms up, 20 reps
B1. BB Skull Crusher
B2. DB Bicep Curls, palms up, both at the same time
Rest 120 seconds.

Set #3. 4 x SD20
Warm-up 20 Cable Curls with bar,
20 DB Triceps Ext behind head
C1. Cable Curls with Rope
C2. Triceps Ext behind head with 1 heavy DB
Rest 120 seconds.
Stretch biceps and triceps.

Training Day #6 Shred Conditioning

Preferably outdoor local football field/track.
Indoor option below if weather doesn't permit.
Warm-up 100 steps Walking Lunges, 50 Lunge Jumps, 3 x
50 yard Sprints 50-70% max speed
20 x 50 yard Sprints, jog back
50 Stadiums
10 x 100 yard Sprints, jog back

Find a trashcan.☺
Stretch quads, hamstrings, and calves.

Training Day #7
Prehab, mobility, flexibility

1. Roll quads individually from knee to hip 20x. Knee to hip, and back to knee is only 1 rep. 20 reps both sides.
2. Stretch both quads, 2 sets of 30 seconds each side.
3. Roll hip flexors. The best way, lay a DB down so it rolls, using the edge of a 10-20 lb. dumbbell, lay on it placing the dumbbell edge just inside your hip bone. Break up the knots.
4. Stretch hip flexors, 2 sets 30 seconds.
5. Roll IT bands, 20 passes knee to hip.
6. Roll lats, 20 passes from very top, down to low back.
7. Stretch lats, 2 sets of 30 seconds.
8. Roll pecs. Lay on top of a 5-15 lb. dumbbell right on chest. Keep arms out wide, make gym angels. This is going to hurt, so suck it up. It will make your chest bigger and fuller looking from the increased range of motion, shoulder width, and blood flow.
9. Stretch pecs doing the doorway stretch on a pole or wall, 2 sets 30 seconds.
10. Roll calves on roller, or handle of a 5-15 lb. dumbbell, 20 passes.
11. Stretch calves, 2 sets 30 seconds.

Done!

Summary

The information that I have shared with you in the first 10 chapters will set you up for massive success and accelerate you towards getting the shredded physique you have always wanted. You have more information, tricks, tactics, hacks, and strategies than anyone else you know. You have 100 times more information than the average personal trainer in America. Achieving the body you want and keeping it month after month, and progressing it continually is a lifestyle.

I recommend that you read this book again immediately, then read it once more. Then read this book once a month to keep yourself in check. Share it with friends. Each time that you read it, you will be reminded of something your forgot. You will pick up something you missed before and it will solidify your knowledge and help you program this information into your mind.

This entire book can be summed up in really just three tips:

1. Nutrition on point seven days a week. Macros!
2. Train hard week after week. Progressively overload!
3. Be consistent and make it a lifestyle.

You do that, and you'll live shredded year-round. That is a promise. My goal is to help as many people around the world as I can to get the shredded body and self-confidence that comes along with it. You deserve it and anyone willing to DTFW deserves it. I have cut a clear path with hacks and all the tricks you need to navigate life and succeed.

Thank you for reading this book. Thank you for your investment. Thank you for learning, applying what you learned, and for becoming a future success story that I know you will achieve. Thank you for sharing this book with the people you care about. Above all, I just want to help the world reach their full potential and live with the wealth of health, confidence, and being shredded. I believe in you. Now go make yourself proud.

Follow us on Instagram @Shredded_Executive
Follow me on social media: @superherostrong
Follow me on Facebook: Daymond Sewall
Feel free to message me anytime with questions.
I'm so proud of this accomplishment.
THANK YOU! **NOW GO DTFW!**

Author Daymond Sewall

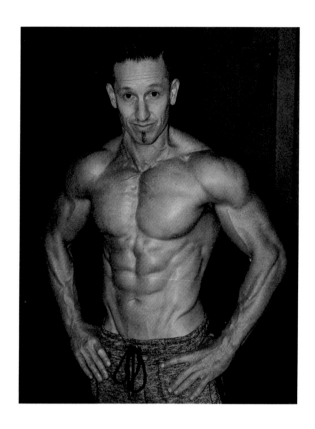

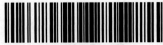